SOMATIC THERAPY WORKBOOK FOR TRAUMA AND STRESS

55+ ILLUSTRATED EXERCISES TO REGULATE YOUR NERVOUS SYSTEM, RELIEVE SYMPTOMS OF STRESS, AND STRENGTHEN YOUR MIND-BODY CONNECTION IN JUST 10 MINUTES A DAY

SARRAH KAYE

Copyright © 2025 by Sarrah Kaye — All rights reserved.

The content contained within this book may not be reproduced, duplicated or transmitted in any form or by any electronic or mechanical means, including information storage and retrieval systems, without direct written permission from the author or the publisher, except for the use of brief quotations in a book review.

Under no circumstances will any blame or legal responsibility be held against the publisher, or author, for any damages, reparation, or monetary loss due to the information contained within this book, either directly or indirectly.

Legal notice:

This book is copyright protected. It is for personal use. You cannot amend, distribute, sell, use, quote or paraphrase any part, or the content within this book, without the consent of the author or publisher.

Disclaimer Notice:

Please note the information contained within this document is for educational and entertainment purposes only. All effort has been executed to present accurate, up to date, reliable, complete information. No warranties of any kind are declared or implied. Readers acknowledge that the author is not engaged in the rendering of legal, financial, medical or professional advice. The content within this book has been derived from various sources. Please consult a licensed professional before attempting any techniques outlined in this book.

By reading this document, the reader agrees that under no circumstances is the author responsible for any losses, direct or indirect, that are incurred as a result of the use of the information contained within this document, including, but not limited to, errors, omissions, or inaccuracies.

Somatic Therapy Workbook for Trauma and Stress

55+ Illustrated Exercises to Regulate Your Nervous System, Relieve Physical Symptoms of Emotional Stress, and Strengthen Your Mind-Body Connection in Just 10 Minutes a Day

By Sarrah Kaye

978-1764076104

To those who have supported me on my healing journey, and to those just beginning theirs—who keep going even when it feels impossible—this is for you.

CONTENTS

A gift for you   xiii
Introduction   xv

1. **THE FOUNDATIONS: UNDERSTANDING SOMATIC THERAPY**   1
   Key Principles of Somatic Therapy   3
   Understanding the Mind-Body Connection: Why Trauma Lies in the Body   4
   Who Might Benefit From Somatic Therapy?   5
   Check Yourself! Is Somatic Therapy Right For You?   6
   Somatic Therapy vs Traditional Talk Therapy   7
   How to Use This Book: A Beginner's Journey   8

2. **THE SCIENCE BEHIND SOMATICS: THE MIND-BODY CONNECTION**   10
   How Trauma Affects the Body   10
   How Stress Affects the Body   12
   The Nervous System: Your Body's Trauma and Stress Response   13
   Understanding Past Trauma   16
   Somatic Symptoms: Recognizing Your Bodies Stress Signals   18
   Your Turn: Noticing the Signals   18
   Persistent Tension   18
   Digestive Disruptions   18
   Unexplained Fatigue   19
   Chest Sensations   19
   Sleep Disturbances   19
   Skin Reactions   20
   Breathing Irregularities   20
   Heightened Sensitivity   20
   Recurring Pain   21

The Role of the Body in Healing Trauma	21
Understanding the Various Approaches in Somatic Therapy	23

3. FIND YOUR INNER BALANCE: SELF-AWARENESS, REGULATION, AND MINDFULNESS — 26

Self-Awareness: Looking Inward and Tuning In	26
Exercise 1: The Three Whys	27
Self-Regulation and Co-Regulation: Balancing Inner and Shared Peace	29
The Self in Control: Exploring Self-Regulation	29
Co-Regulation: The Power of Connection	31
Emotional Regulation: Impact of Emotions on The Body	32
Stress and Anxiety	33
Sadness and Depression	33
Anger and Frustration	33
Joy and Love	34
Shame and Guilt	34
Reaching Your Calm With Emotional Regulation: Exercises	34
Exercise 2: Riding the Wave	35
Exercise 3: Opposite Action	36
Exercise 4: Labeling and Categorizing Emotions	37
The Role of Mindfulness in Somatic Therapy	39
Bringing Presence Into Each Moment: Mindfulness Practices	40
Exercise 5: Mindful Walking	41
Exercise 6: Mindful Eating	42
Exercise 7: STOP Technique	43
Exercise 8: The Body Scan	44
Exercise 9: The Wheel of Awareness Meditation	46

4. LISTEN TO YOUR BODY: SOMATIC AWARENESS AND TRACKING — 51

How to Observe and Track Your Body's Responses	52
Exercise 10: Somatic Tracking for Safety	53

Exercise 11: Somatic Tracking Meditation	54
Releasing Tension: Working With Physical Cues	56
Exercise 12: Palm Pushing	57
Exercise 13: Guided Imagery	57
Exercise 14: 60-Second Somatic Tension Release	60
5. FIND YOUR ANCHOR: GROUNDING TECHNIQUES	**62**
Finding Your Footing With Grounding: Exercises	62
Exercise 15: Sole Connection	63
Exercise 16: Grounding With an Anchoring Statement	64
Exercise 17: Breathe and Press	64
Exercise 18: Nature Walk With Intention	65
EFT Tapping: Releasing Trauma One Tap at a Time	67
Exercise 19: EFT Tapping	68
Why Boundaries Matter: Protecting Your Peace	71
Drawing the Line By Setting Boundaries: Techniques	72
Exercise 20: Toward and Away	73
Exercise 21: Like It/Don't Like It	75
Exercise 22: Exploring Boundaries With Hands	76
6. BREATHE IN, HEAL OUT: THE POWER OF BREATHWORK	**80**
Benefits of Breathwork	81
Harnessing the Power of Breath: Exercises	83
Exercise 23: Diaphragmatic Breathing	83
Exercise 24: Somatic Sighing	84
Exercise 25: Somatic Breath Counting	85
Exercise 26: The Double Inhale Method	86
Exercise 27: Bilateral Stimulation	87
Incorporating Breathwork Into Your Daily Life	88
Exercise 28: The Traffic Light Breath	89
Exercise 29: The Elevator Breather	89
Make a Difference with Your Review	91

7. **BUILD RESILIENCE: RESOURCING AND SEQUENCING** — 92
   - Benefits of Somatic Experiencing® — 94
   - Resourcing: Building Inner Strength and Resilience — 95
   - Tools to Find Stability: Resourcing Exercises — 97
   - *Exercise 30: Five-Step Resourcing* — 97
   - *Exercise 31: How Can I Resource Myself?* — 99
   - *Tips for Using Resourcing Techniques* — 101
   - Sequencing: Mastering the Flow of Sensations — 102
   - *Exercise 32: Sequencing* — 102

8. **HEAL TRAUMA IN SMALL DOSES: PENDULATION AND TITRATION** — 105
   - Pendulation: Shifting Between Comfort and Discomfort — 106
   - What Is Titration? Moving Slowly Through Trauma — 107
   - Exercise 33: Pendulation and Titration — 108
   - *After the Practice* — 110

9. **MOVEMENT AS MEDICINE: YOGA, STRETCH AND SHAKE** — 112
   - Simple Somatic Movements to Try at Home: Somatic Stretching — 113
   - *Exercise 34: Neck Side Stretch (Sukhasana)* — 113
   - *Exercise 35: Bridge Pose (Setu Bandha Sarvangasana)* — 115
   - *Exercise 36: Supine Spinal Twist (Supta Matsyendrasana)* — 117
   - *Exercise 37: Reclined Pigeon Pose (Supta Kapotasana)* — 118
   - Simple Somatic Movements to Try at Home: Somatic Yoga — 120
   - *Exercise 38: Child's Pose (Balasana)* — 121
   - *Exercise 39: Cat-Cow Pose (Marjaryasana to Bitilasana)* — 122
   - *Exercise 40: Seated Forward Bend Pose (Pashchimottanasana)* — 124
   - *Exercise 41: Corpse Pose (Savasana)* — 125
   - Dance, Shake, and Release: Moving Through Emotion — 126
   - *Exercise 42: Shake It Off* — 126

Exercise 43: Dance It Out	128
Qigong: Cultivating Vitality Through Movement	129
Exercise 44: The Gathering Breath	129
Exercise 45: Swaying Tree	131

10. HEAL THROUGH SOMATIC TOUCH: SELF-SOOTHING TECHNIQUES — 133

Benefits of Somatic Touch	134
Somatic Touch in Action: Self-Holding and Self-Soothing Techniques	135
Exercise 46: The Two-Step Self-Holding Exercise	135
Exercise 47: The Gentle Hand Technique	136
Exercise 48: The Rock-and-Breathe Hug	137
The Weighted Blanket Effect	139
Partner Exercises for Safe and Supportive Touch	139
Exercise 49: The Hand Dance	140
Exercise 50: Dynamic Cuddles	141
The Therapeutic Power of Massage	142
Exercise 51: Neck and Shoulder Tension Release	143
Exercise 52: Full-Body Relaxation With a Tool	144

11. RESET AND RESTORE: POLYVAGAL THEORY AND VAGAL NERVE REGULATION — 148

Understanding the Polyvagal Theory	149
The Window of Tolerance	150
Rewiring Relaxation With Vagus Nerve Regulation: Techniques	151
Exercise 53: Tracking Your Nervous System	151
Exercise 54: Expanding Your Window of Tolerance	152
Exercise 55: Progressive Muscle Relaxation (PMR)	154
Expanding Your Somatic Toolkit	155
Using Sound and Vibration to Activate the Vagus Nerve	157
Safe and Sound Protocol (SSP)	157
Humming and Chanting	157
Exercise 56: The Hum Sound	158
Exercise 57: The Voo Sound	158

12. **YOUR 28-DAY SOMATIC THERAPY PLAN** — 161
    Best Tips for Using This 28-Day Plan — 162
    28-Day Somatic Therapy Plan — 163
    Day 1: Foundations of Self-Awareness — 163
    Day 2: Mindful Engagement — 163
    Day 3: Somatic Tracking for Safety — 163
    Day 4: Breath as a Tool — 164
    Day 5: Connecting to the Present — 164
    Day 6: Emotional Regulation — 164
    Day 7: Reflection and Resourcing — 164
    Day 8: Releasing Physical Tension — 165
    Day 9: Grounding in Nature and Self-Touch — 165
    Day 10: Emotional Labeling and Awareness — 165
    Day 11: Deep Sensory Awareness — 165
    Day 12: Emotional Resilience — 166
    Day 13: Vagal Toning and Vocal Activation — 166
    Day 14: Movement for Emotional Flow — 166
    Day 15: Breath Variation and Control — 166
    Day 16: Releasing Tension Through Stretching — 167
    Day 17: Massage-Based Reset — 167
    Day 18: Gentle Somatic Yoga — 167
    Day 19: Qigong-Inspired Grounding — 167
    Day 20: Releasing Resistance — 168
    Day 21: Rebuilding Boundaries and Inner Strength — 168
    Day 22: Self-Support and Stability — 168
    Day 23: Vagal Nerve Regulation — 168
    Day 24: Deep Grounding and Support — 169
    Day 25: Integrating Movement and Breath — 169
    Day 26: Self-Compassion and Healing — 169
    Day 27: Nervous System Closure — 169
    Day 28: Reflection and Looking Ahead — 170
    Making Somatics Work for You — 170
    Morning: Waking Up in a Way That Supports Your Nervous System — 171
    During the Day: Staying Present, Connected, and Balanced — 171
    Evening: Releasing the Day and Resetting Before Sleep — 171

When Old Trauma Responses Sneak In	172
Moving Forward with Somatic Practices	173
Conclusion	175
Bibliography	179

A GIFT FOR YOU

Feeling stiff, tense, or drained after hours at your desk? You're not alone. I've put together **The Somatic Desk Reset**—a simple, effective guide packed with easy exercises to shake off tension, boost focus, and re-energize your body *without ever leaving your chair.*

Want to grab your free copy? Just head over to https://subscribepage.io/lh9v6v or scan the QR code here.

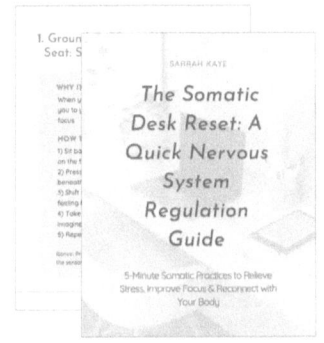

INTRODUCTION

Trauma is a fact of life, it does not, however, have to be a life sentence.

- PETER A. LEVINE

The first time I heard that quote, I froze. Something about it hit differently. Maybe it was because, at the time, I felt like I was stuck in an endless loop of anxiety, searching for something—anything—that gave me hope. Or maybe I just needed to hear that healing was possible, even when my own mind was convinced otherwise. Whatever the reason, that quote stayed with me.

If you're here, I'm guessing some part of this resonates. Maybe stress is making daily life feel heavier than it should be. Maybe anxiety has you wondering if you'll ever feel like yourself again. Or maybe it's something harder to explain—like a pressure in your chest that won't go away or a quiet disconnect from the world. Whatever shape it takes, know this: You're not making it up, and you're not alone.

I've been there. I remember waking up every morning with a weight on my chest I couldn't explain. There was no crisis, no major life event, nothing that *should* have made me feel the way I did. And that was the most frustrating part—I couldn't figure out *why* I felt like this, which meant I had no clue how to fix it. I tried everything I could think of—talk therapy, exercise, mindfulness apps—but nothing seemed to reach the part of me that was hurting the most.

Then, one day, I stumbled across a podcast featuring Peter A. Levine, the founder of Somatic Experiencing®, and Dr. Bessel van der Kolk, author of *The Body Keeps the Score*. They were talking about how the body holds onto unresolved past experiences, how trauma and stress don't just live in your head but get stored in your muscles, your breath, your nervous system. At first, I wasn't sure what to make of it.

But as I continued listening, all those feelings I couldn't explain—the knots in my back, the clenching of my fists, the tears that came out of nowhere—started to make sense. My body wasn't betraying me. It was trying to tell me something, and for the first time, I realized I needed to listen.

That's how I found somatic therapy. A body-based approach to healing that focuses on reconnecting with what's been stored in your body and finding ways to release it. Initially, it felt unfamiliar. I sat quietly, focused on my breath, and noticed what my body had been carrying. It seemed too simple to actually *work*, but slowly, things started to shift. The knot in my back loosened. The weight in my chest lifted. My hands, always clenched into fists, started to relax. And for the first time in a long time, I felt more like *myself*.

If you've tried everything and still feel stuck, somatic therapy might be the missing piece—the tool that reaches the part of you nothing else has. A way to heal rather than just manage what you've been carrying.

I created this workbook to share what I've learned and give you practical, accessible tools for your own journey—no fluff, no complicated theories, just real strategies you can use. A guide to working *with* your mind-body connection, not against it.

Here's what we'll explore together:

- **How trauma, stress, and anxiety leave their mark on your body**—You'll uncover why these feelings often show up as physical sensations, and why they're not "just in your head."
- **Exploring your thoughts, emotions, and behaviors**—Before we explore body-based somatic practices, we'll set the foundations in place by focusing on self-awareness, self-regulation, and mindfulness.
- **Developing somatic awareness**—Trauma, panic, fear, anger, frustration, and depression don't just disappear; they leave their mark, often making you feel stuck, frozen, lost, or even overheated. Through simple, targeted exercises, we'll learn to recognize these signals and work with them instead of feeling caught in their grip.
- **Somatic healing techniques**—We'll use pendulation and titration to gently approach difficult emotions, while introducing resourcing to help you access internal strengths and feelings of safety when needed.
- **Practical tools for nervous system regulation**—Finally, as part of your healing journey, we'll explore breathwork, movement, vagus nerve regulation, grounding, and more as practical tools to release tension, find balance, and reconnect with yourself in a way that feels doable.

And the best part? These aren't just ideas to read about. They are actionable steps and activities you can incorporate into your life. The book will finish with a 28-day plan to help you weave these exercises into your daily routine.

I'll be honest. Healing isn't always a straight line. Some days will be easier than others. But every small step matters, even when it doesn't feel like it in the moment.

By the time you turn the last page of this book, my hope is that you'll feel lighter, freer, and more connected to yourself than you have in a long time. Healing is possible. Peace is possible.

Take a deep breath.

This is the start of something new, and I'm so glad you're here. Let's begin.

1

THE FOUNDATIONS: UNDERSTANDING SOMATIC THERAPY

The mind and body are like parallel universes. Anything that happens in the mental universe must leave tracks in the physical one.

- DEEPAK CHOPRA

SOMATIC THERAPY IS like adjusting a blurry camera lens—you don't realize how out of focus things were until everything sharpens. It shifts your attention to the signals your body has been sending: the way your chest tightens when an old memory resurfaces, the tension in your back during an awkward conversation, or how your shoulders climb when stress sneaks in. These sensations aren't random; they're part of your body's built-in way of processing what's happening beneath the surface.

The word "soma" comes from Greek, meaning "body," but in somatic therapy, it goes beyond what you see in the mirror. It's about experiencing your body from within—tuning into the sensations, movements, and physical tension that shape your experience of the world (Hanna, 2016). Every celebration, argument, and moment of stress leaves an imprint, influencing how you breathe, carry yourself, and even how you feel.

For much of history, therapy focused on the mind, treating thoughts and emotions as if they existed separately from the body. But what happens when the body remembers something the mind can't explain? As researchers and practitioners started to look closer, they found that trauma and emotions settle deep within the body.

Back in the early 20th century, psychoanalyst Wilhelm Reich noticed that his patients weren't just talking about their emotions; they were carrying them, locked up in their muscles like unfinished business (Boadella, 1974). His solution? Breathe deeply to release the tension.

A few decades later, Alexander Lowen expanded on this idea, recognizing that emotions didn't just get stored in the body but actively shaped posture, movement, and breath (Bioenergetic Therapy by Alexander Lowen, 2023). His work made it even clearer: Emotions are felt and embodied.

By the 1970s, somatic therapy started to really take shape. Thomas Hanna introduced the idea of "sensory-motor amnesia," which basically means your brain and muscles stop communicating effectively, often causing chronic pain (Lowndes, 2021). Around the same time, Dr. Peter Levine noticed how animals shake off stress after danger and wondered, "Why don't humans do that?" His curiosity led to Somatic Experiencing®, a method that helps people release the energy trauma traps in their bodies (SEI Communications, 2024).

Others like Ron Kurtz and Pat Ogden built on these foundations, blending mindfulness, neuroscience, and body awareness into practices that help people reconnect with themselves.

Somatic therapy today combines all these ideas—psychology, movement, mindfulness, and cutting-edge neuroscience. While history is fascinating, this book is about what you can actually *do*. In the chapters ahead, you'll find practical techniques to help you reconnect with your body and emotions, creating more balance and ease in your everyday life. Now that you've got the backstory, let's dive into how these principles work in practice.

Key Principles of Somatic Therapy

Let's explore some core ideas that can help you tap into the unique language your body uses to communicate:

- **Listening to the body's signals**: Imagine finishing a long, challenging day—perhaps you had a difficult meeting or a draining conversation. Later, you notice a slight tension in your temples or a subtle tingling in your hands. Rather than brushing these sensations aside, somatic therapy encourages you to consider them gentle nudges from your body, offering clues about what it's processing and what it might need.
- **Creating a safe space for healing**: Picture yourself sinking into your favorite chair after a hectic day, a cozy blanket wrapped around you. That feeling of comfort helps your body relax. For some, this sense of safety might come from the rhythm of steady breathing or the reassuring feeling of your feet firmly on the ground. When you feel secure, your body can ease into healing and release.
- **Tuning into sensations and practicing awareness**: Life has a way of pulling your attention everywhere except your body. You replay a conversation, plan your next move, or scroll endlessly through your phone. During those moments, your body becomes an afterthought. Somatic therapy shifts your focus, asking you to pause and notice. Is there a tightness in your chest? A warmth spreading through your palms? The goal isn't to fix these sensations or make them go away. It's to be curious about them. By sitting with them, even

briefly, you might uncover insights you didn't realize were there.
- **Integrating the mind, body, and emotions**: Your mind, body, and emotions are like musicians in an orchestra. When everything flows, it feels like harmony—your thoughts, feelings, and movements align effortlessly. When something disrupts that flow, though, the harmony can fall apart. Stress might send your thoughts spinning, tighten your chest, and shorten your patience all at once. Somatic therapy helps you recognize these patterns and how each part of you reacts. Like gently retuning each instrument until everything feels balanced again. When this connection is restored, you move beyond just getting through the day—you begin to thrive.

Each of these principles invites you to view your body as a supportive partner on your journey to healing. They not only help you understand what's happening right now but also reveal how past experiences continue to shape your present. Up next, we'll delve into how trauma can settle in the body and why releasing it might feel so challenging.

Understanding the Mind-Body Connection: Why Trauma Lies in the Body

Let's set the scene: You're waiting in line at the grocery store, one hand balancing a basket while you scroll through your phone. Out of nowhere, someone bumps into you. Your heart skips, your shoulders tense up, and your breath catches. They apologize, and you wave it off—it's no big deal, right? But your body didn't get the memo. Even as you move through the checkout line, the tension sticks around, as if you're bracing for something more.

This is your body's way of holding on, even when your mind knows there's no actual threat. Now think about how much deeper that response might go if you've been through something overwhelming or traumatic.

Trauma doesn't just live in your memories—it plants itself in your body because your survival system is designed to protect you, no matter what. When your body senses danger, it doesn't stop to ask questions. Your heart races, your muscles tense, and your senses go on high alert, ready for fight, flight, or freeze—a built-in response that gears you up to confront or escape danger. Ideally, once the danger passes, your body should calm down and reset. But if that resolution never happens, those protective instincts don't fully turn off. They get stuck, leaving your body in a state of constant readiness.

Why does this happen? Your body operates in the now. It doesn't reflect on the past or rationalize the way your mind does. Instead, it reacts to what it senses, carrying forward echoes of danger until it's convinced that you're safe again. That's why trauma can feel so physical—it's not "just in your head." Your body remembers, even when your mind tries to move on.

Rather than urging you to rehash every detail of the past, somatic therapy invites you to simply tune into the present—to notice exactly how your body feels in this moment. The aim isn't to push through or force a resolution, but to create a nurturing environment where your body can naturally begin to release its hold at its own pace.

So, how do you know if this approach is right for you? What should you expect as you get started? Let's talk about it.

Who Might Benefit From Somatic Therapy?

Curious if somatic therapy might be for you? Start by listening to your body. If stress lingers long after the moment has passed or a wave of nerves feels way bigger than the situation, your body might be trying to tell you something. Somatic therapy helps you tune into those signals instead of getting steamrolled by them.

You don't need to be in crisis to benefit from it. Whether you feel stuck, disconnected, or just a little out of sync, this approach helps you get back on speaking terms with your body. It bridges the gap between emotions and physical tension, giving you a way to process what's been lingering and make room for something better.

Check Yourself! Is Somatic Therapy Right For You?

Take a moment to reflect on your experiences and consider these questions:

- **What physical sensations seem to show up in your body, even when you're not sure why?** Think about moments when you've felt a racing heart, tension in your shoulders, or knots in your stomach. What was happening in your life at the time? What do you think your body might have been responding to?

_____
_____
_____

- **If you pause right now to check in with your body, what do you notice?** Close your eyes for a moment and scan your body. Is there any area holding tension, or perhaps one that feels unexpectedly relaxed? What might your body be trying to tell you in this moment?

_____
_____
_____

- **Have you done a lot of personal growth, therapy, or healing work—but still notice physical sensations, discomfort, or patterns that don't quite make sense?** Think about moments where your body reacts (tightens, aches, gets anxious) even though your mind can't connect it to anything specific. Could these be remnants of unprocessed or stored experiences your body is still holding onto? What comes up for you as you reflect on this?

_____
_____
_____

- **What would you like to achieve with somatic therapy?** Is it about healing from past trauma, reconnecting with your body, or creating space for ease and balance?

_____
_____
_____

These questions are here to invite you to get curious and see what comes up. Somatic therapy offers a different way to connect with your experience that goes beyond language. Let's explore how it compares to the traditional talk therapy model.

Somatic Therapy vs Traditional Talk Therapy

Have you ever been in talk therapy, sitting across from someone who's asking you to explain how you feel, but the words just won't come? You know something feels off. Maybe your throat tightens, or there's a strange buzzing under your skin, but how do you explain a sensation? This is where somatic therapy steps in.

Talk therapy is about understanding your story. It helps you unravel the "why" behind your thoughts, emotions, and patterns. Have you ever looked back on an experience and thought, *Oh, so that's why I reacted that way?* Talk therapy helps you turn those moments into clarity, like rereading a book you thought you understood but are now seeing in a whole new way.

But what happens when your body seems to have its own version of the story—one that words can't quite capture? Somatic therapy starts with what your body is already saying. Imagine reflecting on a difficult memory. In talk therapy, you might analyze its emotional impact or unpack how it shapes your behavior. But have you ever paused to notice how that memory feels in your body? Is there a heaviness in your chest? A flutter in your stomach? Maybe your shoulders start to ache. Somatic therapy invites you to ask: Could these sensations be holding pieces of the puzzle you haven't put together yet?

This approach can be especially powerful for experiences that are hard to articulate, like trauma. While talk therapy helps you understand how trauma has shaped your thoughts and emotions, somatic therapy addresses the physical imprints it has left behind. Trauma doesn't just live in your memories; it's stored in your muscles, your breath, and your nervous system. Somatic therapy provides a pathway for your body to release these echoes, completing a cycle that might have been interrupted long ago.

Rather than choosing one approach over the other, think of them as two trusted companions. Together, they create a balance—helping you understand your story while also giving you the tools to rewrite it, not just in your mind, but throughout your whole being.

How to Use This Book: A Beginner's Journey

Where do you start? What steps should you take? This book is here to help you navigate that path.

Somatic therapy, like any new practice, can seem a little abstract at first. You might wonder what it means to listen to your body or how to work with sensations that feel unfamiliar. That's where this book comes in as a companion on your journey.

To make this journey as practical and meaningful as possible, the heart of this book lies in its step-by-step exercises that you can practice in the moment. Each exercise is paired with workbook questions and reflective prompts, helping you analyze the experience and

THE FOUNDATIONS: UNDERSTANDING SOMATIC THERAPY

understand its impact on your body and emotions. You'll also find illustrations for the exercises, offering a clear visual guide so you can follow along and truly connect with what your body needs.

To make things even easier, I've put together a 28-day plan at the end of the book—because let's be real, sometimes knowing where to start is the hardest part. This plan is designed to help you weave these exercises into your daily routine in a way that sticks. Even better? It will only require 10 minutes a day. By the end of the four weeks, you should have a deeper connection with your body, a better understanding of your nervous system, and real, tangible progress.

Whether you're working alongside a therapist or exploring somatic therapy on your own, this book meets you where you are. It's designed to move at your pace, offering a framework that feels both empowering and flexible. These practices are here to help you reconnect with your body and emotions.

No matter where you begin, every moment of attention counts. Healing isn't about rushing toward a finish line; it's about embracing the process and uncovering the wisdom your body has been carrying all along. My hope is that this book becomes your partner in discovering that wisdom, helping you build a sense of balance and ease that's entirely your own.

Let's take this journey together, one moment at a time.

2

THE SCIENCE BEHIND SOMATICS: THE MIND-BODY CONNECTION

You've got a nervous system running the show since day one—regulating everything from your breath to your stress levels, often without you even noticing. But when trauma or chronic stress enters the picture, things don't just go back to normal. Your body keeps score, storing experiences in ways that shape how you feel, react, and move through the world.

Before we can start rewiring those patterns, we need to understand how they got there in the first place. So, consider this your crash course in the mind-body connection—why your nervous system responds the way it does, how it holds onto past experiences, and why some sensations or emotions seem to stick around no matter how much you try to "let it go."

Let's dive in.

How Trauma Affects the Body

Think about your daily commute—whether you're driving or taking public transport. You may find yourself constantly scanning your surroundings, hyper-aware of every horn, sudden movement, or unfamiliar face. It feels like second nature, but it's exhausting, leaving you tense and drained by the time you arrive at your destination. This is how trauma operates within the body, quietly shaping your experience and keeping you on high alert, even in situations that might not warrant it.

Trauma not only disrupts your emotions, it rewrites the way your body operates. One of the most immediate effects is how it impacts your body's natural rhythms. Take your heartbeat, for example. It's meant to rise and fall in response to activity or rest. But trauma can keep it elevated, like a car engine revving in neutral, leading to chronic strain on your cardiovascular system. Over time, this constant state of alertness can increase the risk of heart disease or high blood pressure, even in moments that feel calm (Agorastos & Olff, 2020).

Your body also stores trauma through its stress response system, particularly the hypothalamic-pituitary-adrenal axis (HPA axis). Think of this as your internal alarm system. When triggered, it releases stress hormones like cortisol to help you respond to danger. But trauma can leave that alarm stuck in the "on" position, flooding your body with cortisol long after the threat is gone. This can leave you feeling on edge, disrupt your digestion, and even impair your memory, making it harder to focus or find mental clarity (Center for Substance Abuse Treatment, 2014).

The gut, often called your "second brain," is another place where trauma leaves its mark. You might notice unexplained nausea, changes in appetite, or bloating that seems to come out of nowhere (Leclercq et al., 2016).

The effects don't stop there. Trauma also places significant strain on your immune system. When your body stays in a heightened state of alert, it redirects energy away from immunity to focus on perceived threats. This can leave you more vulnerable to illnesses and persistent inflammation (Forman, 2024). Over time, that inflammation may show as lingering joint pain, fatigue that seems impossible to shake, or autoimmune conditions that flare unpredictably.

Even the way you move can carry traces of trauma. Your muscles might stay tense and this chronic tension can lead to stiffness, back pain, or a sense of physical heaviness (Center for Substance Abuse Treatment, 2014).

These effects aren't just physical; they intertwine with your emotions and daily life. Trauma's imprints can make you feel out of sync, as though your mind and body are speaking different languages. This disconnection can leave you second-guessing your feelings, struggling to trust the signals your body is sending.

Understanding how trauma reshapes your body is essential to understanding why healing takes time. While the brain may logically understand that the danger has passed, the body often lags, trapped in patterns of defense. Recognizing these imprints is the first step toward addressing them, but it's equally important to understand how chronic stress also plays a role in maintaining these patterns.

How Stress Affects the Body

While trauma strikes like a thunderstorm, stress is like a steady drizzle. It might not seem dramatic, but it's equally relentless. Over time, this constant presence seeps into every corner of your life, shaping your mind and body in ways that can feel almost invisible until the effects become too loud to ignore.

Stress is your body's way of preparing for action. Picture rushing to catch a train, navigating a difficult conversation at work, or juggling a to-do list that never seems to end. In these moments, your body responds by releasing stress hormones like cortisol and adrenaline, sharpening your focus and increasing your heart rate. This fight, flight, or freeze response is part of an ancient survival mechanism designed to protect you.

Physically, stress often leaves behind its own set of clues, similar to the manifestations of trauma, such as restless legs at night, tension in your lower back, or persistent fatigue that lingers no matter how much you rest. These aren't random discomforts but signals from your body trying to cope with the demands placed on it. Over time, stress can contribute to chronic conditions like recurring migraines or digestive issues and weaken your immune system, leaving you more susceptible to infections or ongoing inflammation (*Stress Effects on the Body*, 2018).

Instead of resolving and returning to calm, chronic stress keeps your system running on high alert, like an engine idling for hours. Over time, this constant activation wears down your body's ability to maintain balance, leaving you feeling depleted in ways that may not be immediately obvious.

What makes stress so difficult to pinpoint is how easily it blends into daily life. One demanding day might leave you tired, but when those days stack up, the tension becomes part of your routine. The small ways your body adapts—tightening muscles, holding your breath, or staying in a heightened state of awareness—can feel so normal that you don't even notice them.

The emotional impact of stress can be just as significant. Have you ever found yourself snapping at your loved ones over something minor or feeling overwhelmed by a simple task? Stress rewires how you process the world, making even small irritations feel larger (Pietrangelo, 2023). Days filled with this kind of pressure can leave you emotionally drained, heightening anxiety or triggering feelings of helplessness.

The interplay between your mind and body under stress forms a constant loop. A passing worry can trigger physical tension, and that tension, in turn, reinforces a deeper sense of anxiety. This feedback cycle explains why stress can feel so all-encompassing, influencing everything from your thoughts to your energy levels. But why does stress leave such a deep and lasting impact? The answer lies in the nervous system. So, let's jump in and explore how it works.

The Nervous System: Your Body's Trauma and Stress Response

Think of your nervous system as the body's central operations hub, always on the job to protect, regulate, and recover. It not only influences how we experience trauma and stress, but it's also continuously molded by these very experiences. This intricate network, responsible for our reactions, is also where intense experiences are processed and, sometimes, where they settle in ways that affect us long after the event has passed.

To understand how this system manages such high stakes, let's explore its two primary branches: the sympathetic nervous system (SNS) and the parasympathetic nervous system (PNS). The SNS serves as your body's rapid-response team, springing into action when danger feels imminent (Gordan et al., 2015). Imagine walking alone at night and suddenly hearing footsteps behind you. Your heart pounds, your muscles tighten, and your senses heighten. This surge of adrenaline and cortisol activates your body's instinctive toolkit for survival.

However, the same mechanisms that protect you in emergencies can backfire when trauma or chronic stress leaves the SNS stuck in high gear. It's like driving a car with the accelerator pressed down at all times—eventually, the engine wears out. In this state of hyperactivation, you're kept on constant alert while your physical and emotional reserves slowly deplete. Over time, this relentless strain tends to manifest as chronic tension, irritability, persistent headaches, or a racing mind that won't let you sleep (Understand Trauma and the Nervous System, 2023).

The PNS, on the other hand, acts as your body's brake pedal. It's responsible for slowing your heart rate, supporting digestion, and ushering in a sense of calm (Gordan et al., 2015). However, when trauma tips the balance too far, this calming system can overdo it, leading to a state of hypoarousal. In that mode, you might find yourself feeling emotionally numb, chronically tired, or struggling to focus as if the brakes have locked you in place (Mravec, 2006). While this state is meant to conserve energy during overwhelming stress, lingering in it too long can make reconnecting with the world feel like a steep uphill climb.

The interplay between these two systems creates a delicate balance that trauma and chronic stress can quickly disrupt. While the nervous system prepares us to react instantly, the brain steps in to interpret and regulate those responses. A key player in this process is the amygdala—your brain's built-in threat detector—which continuously scans your environment for signs of danger (Bremner, 2006). Imagine sitting in traffic when someone suddenly cuts you off. In that split second, your amygdala fires, activating your sympathetic nervous system to help you respond. Although this rapid reaction is vital in true emergencies, trauma can leave your amygdala overly sensitized, keeping it on constant high alert. As a result, even everyday situations—such as a raised voice or a familiar scent—can trigger the same fight, flight, or freeze response as an actual threat.

Ideally, the prefrontal cortex—the rational part of your brain—should step in to soothe things, reminding you that you're safe now. Unfortunately, trauma often weakens the connection between the prefrontal cortex and the amygdala, letting the latter dominate. This imbalance explains why trauma survivors often feel as if they're reliving their experiences, even when they consciously recognize that the danger has passed (Bremner, 2006).

Trauma can also jumble up your memories, scattering them like puzzle pieces rather than neatly filing them away. Instead of recalling a clear narrative, you might experience flashes—a particular scent, a sudden sound, or a vivid image—that your nervous system treats as if they're happening right now.

Another fascinating player in this story is the vagus nerve—a vital messenger linking your brain to key organs like your heart and gut. Think of it as the body's internal messenger, facilitating communication and helping regulate your stress response. When you take a deep, slow breath, it's the vagus nerve that helps signal to your body that it's safe to relax. We'll talk more about its remarkable role in Chapter 11, where we explore how to unlock its full potential.

Breaking free from these well-worn patterns might seem as challenging as solving a Rubik's cube in the dark, but remember: Healing is built on small, manageable steps. A mindful breath here, a grounding moment there can gently nudge your system back toward balance. Your body isn't working against you—even when it feels that way. Those reactions—the tension, fatigue, racing mind—aren't signs of weakness. They're signals, little messages from within, asking for attention and care.

Before we get lost in today's body chatter, let's rewind the tape for a moment. Think about those times when your body suddenly tenses up or when fatigue hits out of nowhere. Chances are that these responses have deep roots in your past. So, before we decode the latest signals, let's hit pause and explore how your survival strategies came to be. Ready to take a peek back in time? Let's dive into understanding past trauma.

Understanding Past Trauma

We've talked a lot about how trauma shapes the body—how it lingers in muscle tension, breath patterns, and nervous system responses. But understanding trauma in the present is one thing. Looking back and making sense of why you reacted the way you did? That's something else entirely.

Maybe you've wondered why you felt loyalty toward someone who hurt you. Or why you stayed quiet instead of speaking up. Or why keeping the peace always felt more important than standing your ground. Looking back, those patterns might not make sense. But they weren't random, and they weren't your fault. They were your body's way of keeping you safe.

We're used to hearing about fight, flight, or freeze as the go-to survival instinct. But what happens when fighting back isn't an option? Or when leaving would only make things worse? The nervous system has other ways of protecting you.

One such strategy is fawning, a form of survival through agreement. It's like your nervous system quietly saying, "Maybe if I keep things calm, I'll be okay." You might find yourself reflexively apologizing, over-explaining, or people-pleasing—doing whatever it takes to avoid conflict or prevent someone else from getting upset.

Then there's appeasement, which goes a step further. Instead of just dodging harm, you actively work to defuse the threat—smiling through your fear, making yourself useful, and sometimes even aligning with the person causing harm so they see you as non-threatening.

If any of this sounds familiar, it doesn't mean there's something wrong with you. It means your body did exactly what it needed to do to get through. And when survival is on the line, your nervous system isn't worried about how something will look later—it's focused on making sure you stay safe in the moment.

But what happens when those instincts stick around long after the danger is gone? Maybe you still struggle to say no. Maybe you feel uncomfortable when someone's upset, even when it has nothing to do with you. Maybe standing up for yourself feels impossible. That's because your nervous system hasn't gotten the memo that the threat is over. It's still running old survival scripts, even in situations where you don't need them anymore.

And that's where self-blame tends to creep in. You might catch yourself thinking, *Why didn't I do more? Why didn't I fight back?* Survival doesn't always look the way we expect it to. Just because you didn't resist in the way you think you *should* have doesn't mean you weren't strong. Your body did what it had to do to survive and now, you get to learn new ways to move forward.

Researchers like Dr. Stephen Porges have been studying how responses like fawning and appeasement fit into the bigger picture of the nervous system. The science is still evolving, but one thing is clear: our body is wired for survival. Just as it once developed these survival strategies, it's also capable of learning new responses that support trust, safety, and connection.

Now that we've taken a stroll down memory lane and uncovered why your body might have clung to those old habits, it's time to switch gears. The echoes of the past may have shaped your responses, but today your body is sending fresh signals. Let's open that inbox and start reading the messages your body is sending about its current stress and needs.

Somatic Symptoms: Recognizing Your Bodies Stress Signals

Imagine getting an urgent text in a language you don't understand. It's flashing on your screen, insistent, and while it would be easy to ignore, something tells you it matters. Somatic symptoms are like that—signals asking for your attention, not your judgment.

Your Turn: Noticing the Signals

This checklist is a tool to start translating these signals, one by one. As you go through it, try to approach the process with curiosity rather than critique. If something feels familiar, mark it. If it doesn't, move on. There's no pressure to overanalyze or force connections. This is about gently tuning in to what resonates.

Persistent Tension

- ☐ Tight shoulders that feel like they're carrying invisible weights.
- ☐ A jaw that stays clenched even when you're relaxed.
- ☐ A neck that feels stiff every morning, no matter how well you sleep.

Tension in these areas often builds without you noticing, a quiet accumulation of unprocessed stress or emotions.

Digestive Disruptions

- ☐ Nausea that appears before difficult conversations or events.
- ☐ Bloating that seems unrelated to your diet.
- ☐ Sudden appetite changes—eating too much or losing interest in food entirely.

THE SCIENCE BEHIND SOMATICS: THE MIND-BODY CONNEC... 19

These signs show how closely the gut and emotions are linked, with the digestive system mirroring emotional turbulence.

Unexplained Fatigue

- ☐ A sense of exhaustion that lingers, no matter how much you rest.
- ☐ Feeling physically drained after emotionally heavy interactions.
- ☐ A mid-afternoon slump that feels deeper than just needing caffeine.

This isn't about being tired; it's your body working overtime to manage unresolved tension.

Chest Sensations

- ☐ A heaviness in your chest that appears out of nowhere.
- ☐ A fluttering or racing heart during seemingly calm moments.
- ☐ Tightness that makes deep breaths feel difficult.

These sensations are often tied to emotions like anxiety or grief that haven't yet been fully acknowledged.

Sleep Disturbances

- ☐ Struggling to fall asleep because your mind won't stop racing.
- ☐ Waking up in the middle of the night, unable to drift back to sleep.

- ☐ Dreams so vivid they leave you feeling emotionally drained by morning.

Sleep often becomes a battleground for stress, where unresolved thoughts surface and disrupt your rest.

Skin Reactions

- ☐ Acne flare-ups during particularly stressful weeks.
- ☐ Rashes or eczema that seem to have no clear trigger.
- ☐ Itchy patches that appear and fade without explanation.

Your skin often reflects what's happening beneath the surface, reacting to emotional stress just as much as physical irritants.

Breathing Irregularities

- ☐ Shallow breathing that feels automatic in stressful moments.
- ☐ Frequent sighing, as if trying to reset your breath.
- ☐ A sense of breathlessness, even when there's no physical exertion.

These patterns reveal a nervous system that's struggling to find balance.

Heightened Sensitivity

- ☐ Feeling overwhelmed by loud noises or bright lights.
- ☐ Crowded spaces feeling suffocating or draining.
- ☐ A sensitivity to textures or temperatures that didn't bother you before.

These responses point to an overstimulated nervous system, still operating on high alert.

Recurring Pain

- ☐ Headaches that seem to follow moments of high stress.
- ☐ Lower back pain that worsens after emotionally draining days.
- ☐ Aches in your limbs that have no clear physical cause.

These are often how your body expresses unresolved emotions.

As you reflect on the checklist, instead of diving into *why* something feels familiar, just observe what stands out. The goal here is to gently notice patterns emerging without judgment or pressure to find immediate answers.

This process deepens the dialogue you've already begun with your body. The act of marking what feels significant is a quiet and meaningful acknowledgment that your body's signals deserve attention. These signals will become threads you can follow to understand how stress or trauma influenced your physical and emotional state.

While your body may carry the weight of these experiences, it's also the wellspring of healing. Reconnecting with it unlocks a path to restorative, empowering change that's uniquely yours. So, where do you begin? Start by turning your body into an active partner on your journey to healing.

The Role of the Body in Healing Trauma

The body is always working in the background, keeping us alive and functioning, but when it comes to trauma, that quiet resilience becomes essential. Healing doesn't mean erasing the past—it's about learning to carry it differently, so it no longer weighs you down.

One of the most incredible tools for recovery is the brain's ability to adapt. Neuroplasticity—the brain's capacity to rewire itself—offers a way forward, even when old patterns feel inescapable (van der Kolk, 2014). Think of it like a path in the woods: the well-trodden trail may represent the habits trauma has ingrained, but with practice, we can carve out new routes that prioritize safety and resilience. While this transformation doesn't happen overnight, it does happen with consistent, mindful effort.

Sometimes, it starts with something as small as noticing the temperature of your hands. Are they warm? Cool? Somewhere in between? This small act of paying attention engages the brain, creating a moment of focused awareness that might feel insignificant at first, but gradually shifts old patterns—gently steering the brain away from hypervigilance and fostering a deeper sense of calm and presence.

The body also plays a direct role in releasing what trauma has stored. Practices that focus on physical sensations—like mindful movement or grounding exercises—help to reset the nervous system (van der Kolk, 2014). Even things like relaxing a clenched fist or feeling the ground beneath your feet send a quiet, reassuring message to both body and brain: you're safe.

Then there's the power of sensory experiences. Trauma often narrows our focus, shutting out the things that bring us joy or connection. Reintroducing sensory input—a favorite song, the warmth of sunlight, the texture of soft fabric—reminds the nervous system of what safety feels like. These moments aren't just distractions; they help the body relearn how to engage with the present without fear.

But there's more to it than comfort: These sensory experiences tie directly into the brain's ability to change and adapt. When we experience positive sensations paired with calmness, the brain begins to associate those sensations with safety (Forte, 2019). Over time, this helps recondition the nervous system, breaking the cycle of survival-mode responses.

External tools, like medication, can also play a role in recovery. Think of them as a steadying hand—not doing the work for you, but making it easier to find your balance. By easing some of the body's immediate stress responses, medications can help you feel more grounded and open the door to deeper healing practices. If you're considering this option, it's important to connect with the right professionals. Primary care doctors, psychiatrists, or clinical psychologists who specialize in trauma can guide you through understanding how medication might fit into your recovery. They'll help weigh the benefits, potential side effects, and how these tools can support your unique needs.

Reconnecting with the body is a slow, intentional process. There will be moments of progress and moments where things feel stuck. But each step, no matter how small, contributes to the bigger picture. Healing in this context means finding ways to feel at home in your own body again. And when you allow yourself to listen, notice, and engage, the body doesn't just heal—it teaches. It shows you paths to strength and resilience you didn't know were there.

Understanding the Various Approaches in Somatic Therapy

After exploring how the body processes trauma, the natural next question is, "What now?" Somatic therapy offers a range of answers, offering practical ways to release, rebuild, and move forward. Here's a closer look at some of the somatic practices that bring healing within reach:

- **Somatic Experiencing®:** This method helps your body finish the job it started when stress takes over. Instead of letting stress hang around, it gently guides you to notice and release that pent-up energy. Think of it as your body's way of hitting the reset button when it's been stuck in "alert" mode (SEI Communications, 2024).

- **Hakomi Method:** Ever catch yourself crossing your arms when you're feeling a bit vulnerable? This approach invites you to notice those little habits and wonder what they might be saying about your past. It's not about fixing things right away, but about exploring your natural reactions with curiosity and a sense of kindness (Lowndes, 2021).
- **Feldenkrais Method:** If you've ever felt chronic tension or awkwardness in your movements, this method might be for you. It's like giving your body a friendly nudge to try a new way of moving. Through gentle, mindful motions, you can replace old, tense habits with smoother, more comfortable patterns. It's about rediscovering how naturally your body can move, day by day (Lowndes, 2021).
- **EMDR:** Sometimes, memories feel too heavy, and this method helps to ease that load. By using eye movements or alternating sounds, EMDR gently helps your brain reprocess difficult memories so they lose some of their punch. The goal isn't to erase the past but to make it feel less overwhelming (Lowndes, 2021).
- **Alexander Technique:** Ever notice how small habits—like slouching or tensing up while carrying your bag—can cause big discomfort? This approach works on those everyday movements, teaching you to move in a way that feels naturally balanced and free from unnecessary tension (Lowndes, 2021).

You don't have to commit to just one. Many people blend techniques or return to different methods at different points in their healing journey. Whether you need gentle awareness, structured exercises, or hands-on techniques, these approaches offer practical tools to help you reconnect with yourself in a way that feels right.

This chapter has been a foundation—a chance to understand the "what" and "why" behind somatic therapy: Why your nervous system reacts the way it does. Why that tight jaw or restless leg isn't random, but part of a deeper story your body's been telling. Why healing isn't about "fixing" yourself but reconnecting with the signals you may not have realized were there.

Now, we shift from the broader landscape of somatic therapy to the core skills that make everything else possible: self-awareness, self-regulation, and mindfulness. More than just concepts, these are the foundation for real change. Before trying any body-based techniques, you have to first notice what's happening inside you. Moving forward, we'll explore how these skills help you navigate emotions, steady your nervous system, and strengthen your connection to yourself.

3

FIND YOUR INNER BALANCE: SELF-AWARENESS, REGULATION, AND MINDFULNESS

BEFORE WE DIVE into somatic techniques, we're going to be starting with self-awareness, regulation, and mindfulness. Here's why: Somatic work isn't just about doing exercises; it's about *experiencing* them in a way that actually creates change. But if we're disconnected from our emotions, stuck in survival mode, or unaware of what's happening inside us, those exercises might not have the impact they should.

Before we start working with the body, we need to develop the ability to notice what's going on inside us, recognize when we're dysregulated, and have tools to bring ourselves back to balance. This chapter lays that groundwork—so when we get into somatic techniques, you're not just going through the motions, but actually tuning in, feeling the shifts, and creating real change.

Self-Awareness: Looking Inward and Tuning In

Self-awareness is one of those buzzwords that gets tossed around—"At least she's self-aware," people say—but what does it really mean? At its core, self-awareness is about understanding what's going on inside your head—your emotions, thoughts, and behaviors—and how they shape the way you interact with the world. Think of it like having an honest conversation with yourself, where each insight reveals another piece of your inner puzzle. Without that dialogue, you might find yourself simply reacting without knowing why. But with it? You start to recognize the patterns between your thoughts, feelings, and actions, making it easier to choose what actually feels right.

This isn't about obsessing over every reaction or overthinking every moment. Self-awareness is more like noticing you're suddenly snippy after a stressful meeting, or why a certain text from a friend leaves you feeling uneasy. It's not about judging those moments, but about getting curious: What's going on here?

Sometimes, though, we tell ourselves "I'm just in a bad mood," or "It's not a big deal,"—but beneath the surface, there's often something more. If you've ever felt blindsided by your reaction to something, this next exercise can help untangle what's really going on.

Exercise 1: The Three Whys

The Three Whys method is a quick way to get past surface-level answers and uncover the real drivers behind your emotions. It helps you move beyond what you're feeling and toward why you're feeling it.

1. Get a journal or some paper to write down your thoughts on. Think of a situation, decision, or feeling that's been on your mind. It could be something like why you keep putting off responding to a text, or why a certain comment got under your skin.
2. Ask yourself: Why is that? Whatever your first instinct is, write it down—no need to filter or overthink it.
3. Take your answer and ask again: Why do I feel this way? Dig a little deeper. Does this connect to something bigger? A past experience? A belief you hold about yourself?

4. One last time, ask: What's really at the heart of this? By now, you might be surprised at what you've uncovered. If you prefer, you can simply ask "why" again instead. The phrasing isn't what matters—it's the act of gently questioning until you land on something real.

What did you discover? Did your final answer reveal something different than your initial reaction?

_____
_____
_____

It's fascinating to consider that practicing self-awareness actually rewires your brain. There's this framework called S-ART—Self-awareness, Self-regulation, and Self-transcendence—that shows how practices like tuning into your emotions strengthen the rational part of your brain, the prefrontal cortex while calming down the overactive alarm system, the amygdala (Vago & Silbersweig, 2012). Basically, your brain learns to handle stress without flipping out.

An article featuring Vera Ludwig, a research associate at Penn's Platt Labs, found that consistently noticing and acknowledging a behavior can change its "reward value"—meaning the brain stops treating that behavior as inherently satisfying or beneficial (Berger, 2021). Think about mindlessly scrolling on your phone. At first, it might feel like a quick escape, something your brain registers as rewarding. But once you start paying attention—recognizing how it leaves you drained rather than refreshed—the reward value shifts. That behavior no longer feels as satisfying, making it easier to change. In the same way, the more you practice self-awareness, the easier it becomes to shift patterns that no longer serve you.

Self-awareness strengthens your relationships, too. When you understand your patterns, it's easier to communicate what you need, set boundaries, and navigate disagreements without spiraling. Instead of snapping at someone when you're overwhelmed, you can pause, take a breath, and approach the situation with clarity. That steadiness creates room for connection—not just with others, but with yourself.

Noticing what's happening inside you is one thing, but figuring out what to do with it? That's where the real work begins. Self-regulation and co-regulation aren't just helpful—they're essential. They're the tools that keep you grounded when life gets messy and help you stay connected, not only to yourself but to the people around you. Let's explore why these skills matter so much and how they set the stage for everything that follows.

Self-Regulation and Co-Regulation: Balancing Inner and Shared Peace

If self-awareness is like turning on the headlights to see the road ahead, regulation is what lets you adjust the steering when you spot a curve. It's a step further than noticing your emotions or triggers—it's learning to navigate them with intention, using regulation as the tool to course-correct and keep you from getting stuck on autopilot, or veering off track. Self-regulation is the first step in building that steadiness, so let's take a closer look at how it works.

The Self in Control: Exploring Self-Regulation

Let's start with a bit of clarity: Self-regulation isn't about staying calm 24/7—life just doesn't work like that. Instead, it's about building the ability to guide yourself through those moments when things feel out of balance. Self-regulation includes managing your emotions, thoughts, behaviors, and impulses to achieve long-term goals, like cultivating emotional resilience or improving your relationships. Its purpose isn't perfection; it's about developing the capacity to respond intentionally rather than react reflexively.

Picture your nervous system like a pendulum. It naturally swings between alertness and calm throughout the day, adapting to the moment. But stress, frustrations, or even a tiny annoyance can send it swinging too far—leaving you stuck in overwhelm or feeling shut down. Self-regulation is about gently nudging that pendulum back to a steady rhythm, helping you find balance without forcing it.

From a somatic perspective, self-regulation uses body awareness, practical tools, and small mindset shifts to create harmony within your nervous system. Studies show that practices like mindful breathing and body awareness can lower stress hormones, reduce tension, and improve focus (Porges, 2017). Plus, these tools make your nervous system more adaptable, making it easier to bounce back when life throws chaos your way (de Ridder et al., 2012).

The somatic practices we explore in this book will help ease muscle tension or heal physical discomfort but will also help you manage your emotions, thoughts, and behaviors more effectively. We'll be exploring these in more depth throughout the book, but here are a few ways to start strengthening your self-regulation skills now:

- **Mindful breathing:** Your breath is like a reset button you can use anytime. Slowing it down doesn't just calm your emotions—it helps quiet racing thoughts and reduces that jittery, on-edge feeling. Try inhaling for four counts, holding for four, exhaling for four, and holding again for four. It's simple, but it works.
- **Guided visualization:** This one's a little like daydreaming with purpose. Picture a space where you feel completely safe and grounded—maybe it's a quiet beach, a cozy room, or even a memory of a favorite moment. Spend a few minutes soaking in the sights, sounds, and sensations of that place. It's a way to shift your mental focus and settle into a calmer state.
- **Progressive Muscle Relaxation (PMR):** If tension won't budge, PMR helps loosen its grip by tensing and releasing muscle groups, letting your body know it's time to relax. Try this: Start with your toes—squeeze them tight for a few seconds, then release. Then do the same

with your legs, hands, shoulders, and finally, your jaw. With each release, notice the contrast between tension and ease. It's an easy but effective way to help your nervous system settle into a calmer state.

These are just a starting point—simple tools you can use to steady yourself in the moment. However, self-regulation doesn't always have to be a solo effort. Sometimes, finding balance means leaning on the presence and support of others. Let's take a look at co-regulation.

Co-Regulation: The Power of Connection

While self-regulation helps you find calm within yourself, co-regulation reminds us how deeply we're wired for connection. Think about a moment when you felt frazzled after back-to-back deadlines or overwhelmed by a tough conversation. Then a friend calls, and just hearing their steady voice feels like someone turned the volume down on your stress. That's co-regulation in action—the natural way we help each other find stability.

This isn't just a comforting idea; it's rooted in how we're built. From the moment we're born, connection is key to feeling safe. A baby relaxes to the steady rhythm of a parent's heartbeat or the soothing tone of their voice. That need doesn't disappear as we grow—it simply evolves.

Studies show that small acts like holding hands or a simple, reassuring touch can physically lower stress by reducing cortisol levels (Coan et al., 2006). Even shared moments, like breathing in sync or sitting together in silence, can create a powerful sense of calm (Palumbo et al., 2017).

Self-regulation and co-regulation work hand in hand. Some days, using your own tools—a grounding breath, a short walk—is exactly what you need. Other times, leaning on someone else's presence can make all the difference. The real strength lies in recognizing when to look inward and when to reach outward.

Next, we'll zoom in on a specific subset of self-regulation: emotional regulation. While self-regulation takes the broader view of managing your thoughts, behaviors, and impulses, emotional regulation focuses on managing your feelings in real time. Let's explore how mastering this skill can help you navigate those charged moments with clarity and intention.

Emotional Regulation: Impact of Emotions on The Body

Have you ever snapped at someone or completely shut down, only to look back later and think: *What was that about?* Emotions don't just ride shotgun—they're in the driver's seat, and they, of course, affect your body.

Take a moment to reflect on it:

- Think back to a recent moment when you felt a strong emotion—maybe you were annoyed by something, or perhaps you felt unexpectedly happy. Did you notice anything your body was doing in that moment? Maybe a slight change in your breathing, or the way your hands or shoulders felt?

_____

_____

_____

Understanding how your emotions affect your body allows you to give yourself a real-life roadmap to feeling better, both mentally and physically. When emotions run wild, they trigger immediate reactions and can leave lasting imprints on our health. Here's a friendly rundown of how different emotions can show up in your body.

Stress and Anxiety

- Your heart starts beating fast while your muscles tense up like you're about to sprint.
- That constant "on" mode lowers your energy and leaves your immune system feeling a bit deflated.
- Before you know it, this uninvited hyper-alertness can edge you toward anxiety or even depression (Neacsiu et al., 2018).

Sadness and Depression

- Fatigue settles in, making everything feel heavier—like moving through water.
- Your appetite might swing wildly, pulling you toward comfort foods or making meals feel like a chore (Neacsiu et al., 2018).
- Over time, these lingering blues can dull your energy, disrupt your sleep, and leave your body feeling out of sync (Lumley et al., 2011).

Anger and Frustration

- A surge of adrenaline floods your system, leaving you tense, wired, and on edge.
- That tension often lands in your jaw, shoulders, or stomach, bringing headaches, digestive issues, or muscle pain (Neacsiu et al., 2018).
- If anger keeps building, it can start to take a toll on your heart and overall well-being (Lumley et al., 2011).

Joy and Love

- Your whole body softens as stress fades into the background.
- A sense of warmth and ease washes over you, slowing your breath and relaxing your muscles (Cherry, 2024).
- These feel-good moments do more than lift your mood—they boost your immune system, support heart health, and build long-term resilience (Cherry, 2024).

Shame and Guilt

- A wave of stress hits, making you overly self-conscious—like all eyes are on you.
- Your muscles tighten, especially in your chest and stomach, making it feel like you're carrying extra weight (Leary, 2015).
- Over time, that heaviness can wear you down, throwing off digestion and making it harder to shake feelings of self-doubt (Lumley et al., 2011).

This rundown shows not only how emotions can play tricks on your body in the moment, but also exposes the lasting impact they can have if left unchecked.

Now that you've begun to identify how emotions arise within you, it's time to take the next step: exploring how to respond. Emotional regulation comes alive when you learn to release emotions safely and cultivate the strength to meet whatever comes your way.

Reaching Your Calm With Emotional Regulation: Exercises

The exercises ahead are designed to guide you through engaging with your emotions in ways that feel safe and empowering. There are no rules—you can adapt them to suit what feels right for you and your body in the moment. You get to choose what works, refine it, and make it your own.

Exercise 2: Riding the Wave

"Riding the Wave" is all about letting emotions run their course without letting them knock you over. Think of it like riding an ocean wave—when you fight a strong one, you're more likely to get pulled under. But if you move with it, you stay afloat. The same goes for emotions. When you resist or try to shut them down, they tend to stick around longer, often showing up as stress or tension in your body. Letting yourself feel and flow with them not only makes them less overwhelming but also helps your nervous system build resilience.

Now, let's give it a try:

1. Sit comfortably in a quiet space where you feel safe and won't be interrupted.
2. Name what you're feeling. Saying it aloud or writing it down brings clarity—"I'm frustrated" or "I'm overwhelmed."
3. Picture the emotion as a wave building in strength. Instead of fighting it, imagine floating with it, trusting that it will subside.
4. Focus on where the emotion shows up in your body. Is it a tingling in your fingertips or a sudden chill in your body? Avoid judging these sensations—just notice them.
5. Remind yourself that emotions, like waves, are temporary. As the intensity fades, gently shift your focus back to the present.

Take a look at the wave illustration below. Use it to track the rise and fall of your emotions. Start by marking where you are right now

—climbing, peaking, or subsiding—and jot down what you're experiencing in your body during that phase.

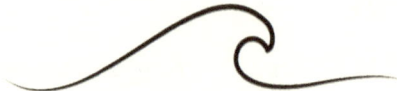

- How does this wave feel to you? Write a sentence or two describing the emotions or sensations you're experiencing at this moment—consider its tone, intensity, or the way it moves through you.

_____
_____
_____

Exercise 3: Opposite Action

When emotions pull you toward unhelpful behaviors—like snapping at someone when you're angry or isolating yourself when you're sad—opposite action helps you choose a new path.

Now, it's your turn to try it:

1. Notice what your emotion is pushing you to do. Does anxiety make you want to avoid a task? Does sadness make you want to withdraw?
2. Act intentionally in a way that counters the emotional impulse. For instance, if frustration makes you want to yell, try speaking calmly. If you feel like isolating, reach out to a friend or take a walk.
3. Follow through with your opposite action, even if it feels awkward at first.

Now that you've tried an opposite action, take a moment to reflect on how it felt. Let's break it down together:

- What emotion were you experiencing at that moment? What was your first instinct—what did you want to do?

_____
_____
_____

- What opposite action did you choose to try instead? Did it change how you felt, even slightly?

_____
_____
_____

Exercise 4: Labeling and Categorizing Emotions

Sometimes emotions feel like a tangled mess—big, overwhelming, and hard to figure out. But when you take the time to name them, their intensity starts to ease. Labeling an emotion turns it from something vague and unsettling into something you can understand and work with. Once you know what you're dealing with, you can decide what to do about it.

Let's break it down step by step:

1. Use the emotion wheel below to explore what you're feeling.
2. Start with the core emotion. Are you feeling angry, worried, or excited? Place your finger on the corresponding section of the wheel.

3. Dive deeper into the wheel to pinpoint the nuance. For example, if you're feeling anger, is it closer to frustration or resentment? If you're sad, is it disappointment or grief?
4. Reflect on the trigger. What do you think sparked the emotion—a conversation, an event, or maybe a thought?
    o _____
5. Name the emotion aloud or write it down. Giving it a name helps turn an abstract sensation into something tangible and manageable.
    o _____

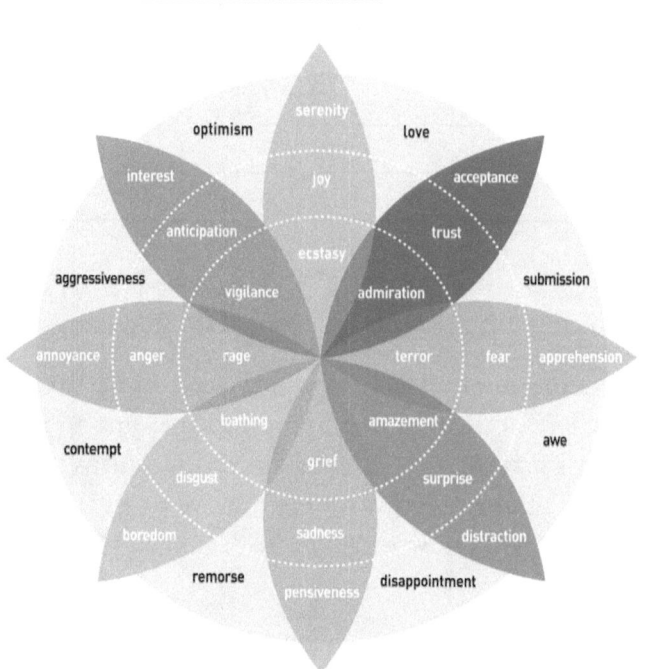

As you explore the emotion wheel, use the table below to track your findings. This will help you better understand your emotions and how they show up in your body:

Emotion	Trigger	Body sensation

Revisit the wheel whenever you need to check in with yourself. The table is a great way to reflect on your patterns, how emotions manifest in your body, and what might be influencing them.

As you try out these exercises, you'll start to notice they do more than just help you handle emotions—they give you a sense of stability when things feel messy. Over time, they'll become less like tools you have to think about and more like natural habits that guide you through the highs and lows. One powerful way to deepen that steadiness is mindfulness.

The Role of Mindfulness in Somatic Therapy

When life feels overwhelming, mindfulness offers a soft place to land: the present. Not the endless loop of yesterday's "what ifs" or tomorrow's "what nows," but the right here, right now. In the world of somatic therapy, psychologist Yevhenii Lozovyi (2023) calls this approach "Embodied mindfulness." Instead of letting your thoughts hog the spotlight, this practice gently nudges you to tune into your body: the steady rhythm of your breath, a little tension in your shoulders, or the satisfying way your chest expands when you're relaxed. By building this kind of awareness, you sharpen your self-regulation skills, catching those early hints of stress before they escalate into full-blown overwhelm.

Mindfulness isn't a modern invention. For thousands of years, traditions like Buddhist meditation emphasized awareness and presence as central to balance and harmony. But it wasn't until the 1970s that mindfulness entered the scientific spotlight. Dr. Jon Kabat-Zinn, a professor of medicine, adapted these ancient practices into Mindfulness-Based Stress Reduction (MBSR), creating a structured approach that revealed mindfulness's potential for reducing stress and improving overall mental health (Keng et al., 2011).

Since then, research has reinforced mindfulness's benefits. Studies consistently show that those who practice mindfulness regularly report lower stress and anxiety levels (Hofmann et al., 2010). Even more, it alters how the body responds to pressure, calming the nervous system, improving focus, and reducing emotional reactivity (Pascoe et al., 2017). These findings underscore mindfulness as a powerful tool for cultivating clarity and balance amidst chaos.

That said, mindfulness isn't always easy. Some days, your mind is racing, your to-do list keeps growing, and it feels like you've got a hundred tabs open at once. But mindfulness doesn't expect you to shut it all down or force yourself into instant calm. It encourages you to take small steps: noticing the coolness of a glass of water, the rhythm of your breathing, or the sunlight filtering through a window. Each small moment builds your capacity to be present, even when it feels hard.

Let's dive into some simple ways to practice mindfulness and experience how these small shifts can lead to meaningful, lasting change.

Bringing Presence Into Each Moment: Mindfulness Practices

Mindfulness invites you to see your everyday moments in a new light. Let's explore a few simple ways to bring that presence to life.

Exercise 5: Mindful Walking

You might think, "Walking? Isn't that just... walking?" But hear me out—what if those steps could do more than just take you somewhere? What if they could pull you back to the present, quiet your mind, and anchor you in the here and now? It's about making the steps you already take mean something more.

Let's see how:

1. Choose a path where you feel comfortable—maybe it's the sidewalk in your neighborhood where the trees arch overhead, a park with the sound of birds in the background, or even a familiar stretch of your backyard—somewhere you can settle into the rhythm of walking.
2. As you begin, focus on the sensation of your feet meeting the ground. How does it feel underfoot? Notice the texture, like soft grass, firm pavement, or crunchy leaves.
3. Tune into the world around you. Can you hear the shuffle of your footsteps, a car passing in the distance, or maybe the hum of nearby life? What about the air—does it carry the smell of fresh laundry, damp soil, or someone's weekend barbecue?
4. Let your breath join the rhythm of your steps. Try inhaling for three steps and exhaling for three. If it feels forced, let your breath settle into its own pattern and simply notice it.
5. When your thoughts wander (as they will), gently return your focus to the movement of your body or a sensation, like the breeze against your face.
6. As you finish, pause and reflect. Take a moment to appreciate the time you've spent grounding yourself in the present.

After your walk, write down or think about the most vivid sensations you experienced:

- Was there a moment when you felt particularly present? What made that stand out?

_____
_____
_____

- How might you carry that awareness into the rest of your day?

_____
_____
_____

Exercise 6: Mindful Eating

How often do you really pay attention when you eat? Most of us barely notice our meals as we scroll through our phones, rush through lunch, or zone out in front of the TV. Eating can end up feeling like just another task on the to-do list instead of the nurturing, nourishing experience it's meant to be. What if, instead, you turned eating into an act of self-care? Mindful eating invites you to slow down, savor each bite, and truly connect with the food in front of you.

Here's how you can bring a little more presence to the table:

1. Start by removing distractions like phones or screens. Choose a calm space to enjoy your meal.
2. Before taking a bite, take a moment to observe your food.

Notice its colors, textures, and aromas. Reflect on its journey—from growth to preparation.
3. With your first bite, fully engage your senses. What do you taste? How does it feel in your mouth—crunchy, smooth, warm, or cool?
4. Chew slowly, savoring each moment. Notice how the flavors shift or deepen as you continue.
5. Pause between bites. Set your utensil down and take a breath. Let yourself fully experience each bite before moving to the next.
6. As you eat, check in with your body. How full do you feel? Are you satisfied, or are you eating out of habit?

Use the questions below to reflect on the experience:

- What did you notice about the taste, texture, and aroma of your meal?

_____

_____

_____

- How did slowing down affect the way you experienced your food? Did it change how much you enjoyed it?

_____

_____

_____

Exercise 7: STOP Technique

Picture this: Your brain's juggling five tabs at once—emails, errands, and that thing you were supposed to remember but forgot. Everything feels tangled, and your chest tightens with the pressure. This is where the STOP Technique steps in. It's a great way to hit "pause" on the chaos to catch your breath and get back to yourself.

Let's break it down:

1. **S**: Stop what you're doing. Take a moment to pause.
2. **T**: Take a breath. Inhale deeply and exhale slowly, letting yourself settle.
3. **O**: Observe your experience. What thoughts, emotions, or physical sensations are present? What's happening around you?
4. **P**: Proceed with intention. Choose your next action mindfully, whether that's continuing what you were doing or shifting gears.

Once you've tried the exercise, think about where it fits into your day.

- When might the STOP Technique help you pause and reset? Write down a few situations:

_____
_____
_____

Exercise 8: The Body Scan

Throughout the day, tension has a way of creeping in quietly. Maybe it starts with your shoulders lifting slightly during a stressful email or a faint ache in your lower back after sitting for too long. These sensations are often easy to ignore until they get louder. Body scanning helps you catch those signals earlier. It's like shining a flashlight over different parts of your body, noticing what's there without judgment.

. . .

Now, let's try it out:

1. Find a quiet space where you won't be disturbed. Sit or lie down in a comfortable position that supports relaxation. Close your eyes or soften your gaze, letting your focus turn inward.
2. Take a few deep breaths. Feel the air moving in through your nose, filling your chest or belly, and leaving as you exhale. Let this rhythm anchor you to the present moment—it's your safe place to return to if your mind starts to wander.
3. Gently shift your attention to the top of your head. Notice any sensations there—warmth, tingling, or even nothing at all. Let yourself observe without trying to change anything.
4. Gradually bring your attention to each part of your body. Spend a few moments noticing what's present in your:
    - **Face and jaw:** Are your jaw and forehead relaxed or tight? Do you feel warmth or tension?
    - **Neck and shoulders:** Are they heavy, stiff, or neutral?
    - **Arms and hands:** What sensations are present in your upper arms, forearms, palms, and fingers? Do you feel any warmth, tingling, or tightness?
    - **Chest and back:** Feel the rhythm of your breath. Is there tightness, ease, or something else in your chest or back?
    - **Abdomen:** Does it feel soft, tight, or relaxed?
    - **Hips and legs:** Tune into your hips, thighs, knees, calves, ankles, feet, and toes. Do you notice a sense of pressure, lightness, or maybe a soft pulsing?
5. Describe the sensations you feel in each area to yourself: Are they sharp, dull, warm, cool, or neutral? If your

mind drifts (and it will), gently return to the part of your body you were focusing on.
6. Once you've moved through each part, bring your attention to your body as a whole. Notice how it feels to connect with yourself in this way—grounded, present, or maybe even more relaxed.

After finishing the body scan, take a moment to reflect on what you noticed:

- Was there a body part that surprised you with how much attention it needed? What might that mean for how you carry tension or stress?

_____
_____
_____

- Did your overall awareness change as you moved through your body? Did you feel more connected, disconnected, or something else?

_____
_____
_____

Exercise 9: The Wheel of Awareness Meditation

Imagine your mind as a wild storm—winds howling, lightning flashing, and thunder shaking everything around you. Thoughts whip by like debris, emotions surge like tidal waves, and sensory experiences come at you like a torrent. If you have 20–30 minutes to slow down and check in with yourself, this meditation offers a way to step back from the noise and take in the full picture. The Wheel of Awareness by Dr. Dan Siegel (2018) helps you tune into different layers of your experience—your senses, body, thoughts, and connections—all while staying grounded in the present.

Let's try it out:

1. Find a quiet space where you won't be interrupted. Sit comfortably or lie down if that feels better. Keep your spine relaxed but upright, hands resting naturally. Close your eyes or soften your gaze, letting your focus settle.
2. Take a few deep, natural breaths. Feel the rise and fall of your chest or belly, letting the rhythm of your breath anchor you.
3. Now, refer to the wheel here—at the center is the "hub," representing your core awareness, and around it, are four "quadrants," each offering a different window into your experience. We'll take a few moments in each one:
    - **The first five senses:** Tune in to what's happening around you. Notice the sounds in the room, the temperature on your skin, and any lingering tastes or scents. If your eyes are closed, you might briefly open them to take in your surroundings before closing them again. What stands out? What's subtle? Just observe.
    - **The sixth sense (Interoception):** Shift your awareness inward. Slowly scan from head to toe, noticing sensations—warmth, tingling, heaviness, ease. No need to analyze, just observe what's present.
    - **The seventh sense (narrative/thought):** Now, turn to your mind. What thoughts drift in? What emotions show up? Let them pass like clouds, noticing them without getting pulled in. Is there a pattern? A familiar storyline? Just watch.
    - **The eighth sense (Connection/Interconnectedness):** Finally, bring your focus to connection.

Not just with people but with the world around you. You might think of someone who brings you comfort, feel the presence of nature, or sense your place in something larger. Notice any warmth, belonging, or even resistance that comes up. Stay here for a few breaths.

4. Now, return your focus to the hub of the wheel—your core awareness. Rest here for a moment, simply noticing that you're aware of all these experiences without being swept away by them.

5. When you're ready, bring your focus back to your breath. Take a few deep inhales and exhales, then slowly open your eyes. Carry that steadiness with you as you move forward.

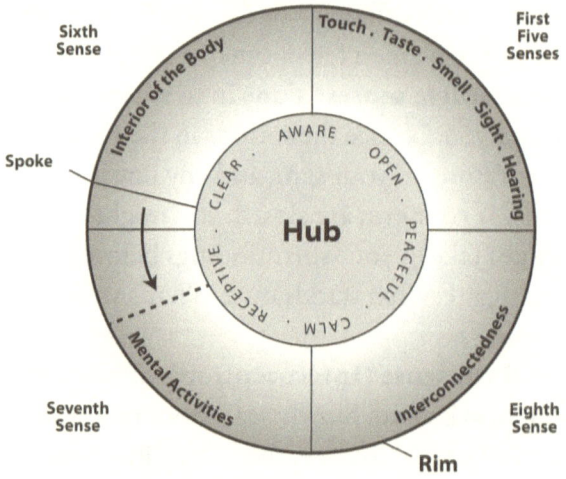

After your meditation, take a moment to reflect:

- Which part of the meditation felt the most natural? Which part felt challenging?

- What surprised you about what you noticed?

At first, these exercises might feel like conscious efforts—steps you have to plan or remind yourself to take. But over time, they start to fit naturally, like finding your footing on a well-worn path. Mindfulness becomes less about setting time aside and more about how you move through your day—a quiet, steady presence in everything you do.

Picture your day as a series of tiny windows, each offering a moment to pause and tune in. These windows don't demand an hour of quiet or a secluded retreat—they're already part of your routine. It might be the stillness before your first sip of coffee, noticing the warmth of water cascading during a shower, or even the lull at a red light. Each window invites you to breathe, notice, and reconnect, even if it's just for a few seconds.

The key to incorporating mindfulness is to start where you are. Every time you pause to notice your breath, name a feeling, or bring curiosity to a sensation, you're reinforcing your connection to yourself. Every attempt is evidence of how you show up for yourself—messy, human, and wholeheartedly trying.

But this is just the beginning. Finding your balance opens the door and somatic awareness invites you to walk through it. As we move into the next chapter, we'll explore somatic awareness and tracking, a practice that helps you decode the signals your body has been quietly (or not so quietly) sending all along. What stories has your body been holding onto, waiting for you to notice? Let's explore what happens when you truly start to listen.

4

LISTEN TO YOUR BODY: SOMATIC AWARENESS AND TRACKING

Before we dive into the somatic practices that can help you navigate trauma or chronic stress, we need to hit pause and talk about somatic awareness. It's what allows you to recognize and understand the signals your body is sending before you can work with them. Like seeing the sky darken before the storm hits, it helps you understand what's coming and how to move through it. Without it, those practices might feel like random moves. With it? You become fluent in your body's language, ready to respond with intention and care.

This isn't the kind of awareness that we explored in the last chapter. It's deeper and more immediate. Think about a moment of frustration, like after a difficult commute. General self-awareness might help you recognize that you're annoyed, but somatic awareness asks a different question: Where does that frustration live in your body?

Here's why this matters: Studies show that paying attention to your body's signals doesn't just help you understand what you're feeling—it actually makes emotional processing smoother and improves overall well-being (Keng et al., 2011). When you tune into sensations, you're giving your body the acknowledgment it needs to reset and regulate itself.

But it's more than just syncing up with your inner rhythm.

Somatic awareness rewires how you fuel your recovery. Here's what that transformation looks like:

- **Release that's genuine, not forced:** Think about when you've held tension in your shoulders for so long that you forgot it was there. Somatic awareness allows you to meet tension with curiosity, not force. Maybe rolling your shoulders or just noticing the tightness helps it soften, showing you how release often comes when it's ready—not when it's pushed.
- **Building trust in your body:** Over time, you'll expect a certain body sensation or reaction in certain situations, and it won't scare you because you'll know exactly why it's there.
- **Resilience in action:** Life's uncertainties don't disappear, but somatic awareness helps you navigate them. Tuning into your body lets you sense when you're nearing burnout or when you're ready to take on more. It helps you adapt rather than react.

Once you've started noticing and naming what's happening in your body, the natural next step is figuring out how to respond. That's where somatic practices step in as a hands-on way to interact with those signals. These practices give you the tools to work through what your body's carrying, whether it's the weight of today's stress or something that's been lingering for much longer. To make sense of it all without overcomplicating things, let's dive into tracking as a way to decode what your body is trying to tell you.

How to Observe and Track Your Body's Responses

Imagine for a moment that your body is a dance floor and every sensation—big or small—is a dancer moving across it. Some are light and graceful, others stomp their feet, demanding your attention. Your job? Not to judge the dancers or scramble to clear the floor. It's to watch the movements, notice the patterns, and see how they shift with the rhythm of your day.

This kind of mindful observation is what turns somatic awareness into something deeper. You're no longer just noticing that your neck feels stiff or that your hands are restless. You're beginning to map these sensations, tracing where they come from, how they change, and what helps them ease.

Unlike a full-body scan, which methodically checks in with every part of your body—like turning on the lights in every room to get a full picture—somatic tracking hones in on one specific sensation, allowing you to explore it with curiosity. So, let's try some practical tools to start tracking your body's responses.

Exercise 10: Somatic Tracking for Safety

Imagine you're sitting at a cozy coffee shop, sipping your favorite latte, or maybe you're at your desk trying to finish up some work. Then, out of nowhere, that familiar discomfort—pain, tension, or even anxious thoughts—starts to creep in. Instead of pushing it away or ignoring it, what if you paused and gave it some curious attention? This exercise helps you explore those sensations in a way that reassures your brain you're safe, even when the discomfort shows up.

1. When you notice the discomfort, pause whatever you're doing. Whether it's sipping your coffee or typing away at your desk, take a moment to sit back and focus.
2. Observe the sensation with curiosity, as if you're studying something new. Is it sharp, dull, or pulsing? Does it shift or stay still? Try to approach it with a sense of exploration, noticing without getting caught up in the emotions that come with it.
3. Accept the sensation for what it is: just your body sending signals. Say to yourself, "This is temporary. It's just a thought or neurons firing."

4. Reassure yourself with kind, grounding words: "This is not harmful, and I am safe. My body knows how to handle this."
5. Let the moment pass naturally. Remind yourself, "I don't have to fix this right now. My body is strong, and I'll be okay."

Take a few deep breaths and notice any shifts in how you feel. To track your experience, use the table below to capture what you noticed during the exercise:

What's the sensation	How it felt	How it changed over time	What I felt afterward

Exercise 11: Somatic Tracking Meditation

If you love a calming practice that combines mindfulness with body awareness, this one's for you. Somatic tracking meditation helps you approach discomfort or pain with curiosity, allowing your brain and body to relax into a state of safety.

1. Find a quiet, comfortable spot where you can sit or lie down without distractions. Let your body settle into the space, allowing your shoulders to drop and your hands to rest naturally.

2. Take a few deep breaths, starting with an easy rhythm like inhaling for three seconds and exhaling for three. Let your breath lengthen as you begin to relax.
3. Set the intention to explore any discomfort or tension in your body. Observe with openness.
4. Focus your attention on an area where you feel pain, tension, or discomfort. Imagine the sensation as a curious object in a museum, something to study rather than fear. If no discomfort is present, try a gentle movement to create mild tension for exploration.
5. Invite the sensation to unfold. Let it do whatever it needs to without trying to change or control it. Notice shifts in intensity, texture, or location, like warmth, tingling, or tightness.
6. If emotions like anxiety or sadness arise, notice where they show up in your body. Offer the same curious attention to these sensations, letting them be without resistance.
7. When ready, shift your focus to a part of your body that feels good—perhaps a warm spot, a soft tingling, or an area of ease. Stay here for a few moments, letting these sensations ground you.
8. Gently transition out of the meditation by returning your focus to your breath or noticing the sounds around you. Let your awareness expand to the room before moving on with your day.

After the meditation, take a moment to reflect:

- What sensations stood out the most, and how did they change?

_____
_____
_____

- What did you notice when you observed without trying to change anything? Did anything feel different?

_____
_____
_____

- Which part of your body felt calm or safe, and how can you connect with that feeling throughout your day?

_____
_____
_____

These exercises are windows into your body's story. As you practice, you begin to see the patterns: where tension gathers, how it shifts, and what helps it ease. This growing awareness is the first step toward healing—it's about getting curious, paying attention, noticing what helps, and learning to trust the signals your body sends.

With these patterns starting to take shape, the next step is clear: How do you respond to what your body is asking for? This is where we turn awareness into action and learn how to release tension in ways that support your body's natural balance.

Releasing Tension: Working With Physical Cues

Tension in your body is a lot like the atmosphere in a room when a conversation stops abruptly—you might not notice it building, but once it's there, it's hard to ignore. It lingers quietly, settling into your muscles until suddenly, it's all you can feel.

Your body is built to reset and find balance, but long days, stress, and everyday frustrations can jam that natural reset button, leaving tension stuck like static on an old radio. The good news? You can

LISTEN TO YOUR BODY: SOMATIC AWARENESS AND TRACKI... 57

tune back into a clearer signal. Here are some simple techniques to release that buildup and bring ease back into your day.

Exercise 12: Palm Pushing

Some days, tension feels like static buzzing through your body, too much energy with nowhere to go. Palm pushing offers a focused way to release that energy while grounding yourself in the present.

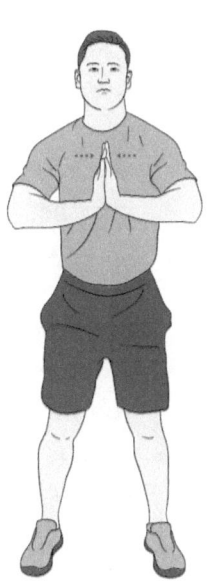

1. Sit or stand with your feet firmly planted.
2. Press your palms together at chest level, applying gentle but firm pressure.
3. Hold the push for 5–10 seconds, noticing the effort in your arms and chest.
4. Release, letting your hands relax at your sides.
5. Repeat 3–5 times, focusing on the sensations of tension building and releasing.

- What did you notice as you created and released pressure? Did it help ease some of that built-up tension?

_____

_____

_____

Exercise 13: Guided Imagery

Guided imagery is like giving your mind and body a moment to step into a place where stress can't follow. This practice is especially helpful when your thoughts won't slow down, when you're running on empty, or when you just need a moment to reset. Letting yourself sink into a peaceful scene can be a simple way to quiet the chaos and come back to yourself.

1. Find a comfortable spot to sit, letting your body settle. Take a few deep breaths, allowing each exhale to soften your shoulders, your jaw, or anywhere you've been holding tightness.
2. Close your eyes, and let's step into a forest together. A winding trail stretches ahead, lined with soft moss and dappled with sunlight filtering through the tall trees above. The air is crisp, almost electric like it's just been refreshed by the morning dew.
3. As you walk, notice the ground beneath you. Maybe the moss feels springy, or the crunch of leaves adds a satisfying sound to each step. Your body feels steady and grounded, as though the forest floor is gently holding you with every movement.
4. Listen closely. The breeze moves through the trees, their leaves rustling like a quiet conversation. A waterfall flows in the distance, its steady rhythm filling the air, while a bird nearby adds its own little melody.
5. Pause for a moment. Reach out and brush your hand against the rough bark of a tree, feeling its cool, sturdy texture. Run your fingertips along the velvety edges of a fern, letting the sensation remind you to slow down and simply feel.
6. Stay here as long as you need, letting the sights, sounds, and textures of the forest surround you like a comforting embrace. Let the rhythm of the forest become your rhythm, soothing any tension in your body.
7. When you're ready, take a deep breath and gently guide yourself back to the present. Open your eyes and notice

the world around you, carrying some of that forest calm with you into the rest of your day.

Let's pause for a moment to explore how this experience felt for you:

- What part of the forest imagery felt the most vivid—was it the sounds, textures, or colors?

_____
_____
_____

- What changed in your body as you focused on the sensations? Did your shoulders relax, your jaw unclench, or maybe your breath felt a little lighter?

_____
_____
_____

- How do your body and mind feel now compared to before the exercise?

_____
_____
_____

This forest, beach, or anywhere that feels right is yours to return to whenever you need a break. Let it remind you that peace is always within reach.

Exercise 14: 60-Second Somatic Tension Release

Sometimes tension creeps in without us even noticing and this quick somatic release uses simple, mindful movements to help your body let go of what it's holding onto, leaving you feeling lighter in just one minute.

1. Let your teeth part and feel your jaw loosen. Exhale slowly and notice the tension melt away.
2. Bring your shoulders down and gently roll your neck from side to side like you're drawing a smile with your chin.
3. Stretch your fingers wide, then let them go limp. Give your hands a little shake, like you're shaking off water.
4. Slowly move your eyes in a full circle, then shift them from side to side. Blink a few times to reset.
5. Open your mouth wide and stretch your tongue out as far as it'll go. Let your face relax—drop your jaw, soften your cheeks, and ease your forehead. Hold for a few seconds, then gently close your mouth and return to neutral.
6. Place one hand on your stomach and take a deep breath in, letting your belly expand fully. Exhale slowly, as if you're blowing out a candle.

Now that you've gone through the movements, let's figure out what worked best for you. Use the table below to note how each movement felt, and which ones made the biggest difference:

Movement	How effective was it? (1-5)	Why it helped (or didn't)
Unclenching jaw		
Dropping shoulders		
Rolling neck		
Stretching fingers		
Shaking hands		
Rolling eyes		
Sticking out tongue		
Belly breathing		

As you fill in the table, think about what felt easiest or most satisfying. Maybe your shoulders instantly relaxed, or shaking out your hands felt like shaking off a bad day. Keep this as a quick reference to guide you the next time you need a fast tension release.

These exercises can become part of how you move through life—a way to tune in, reset, and reconnect. As they integrate into your daily rhythm, tension might start to feel less like a problem to solve and more like a signal guiding you toward balance.

In the next chapter, we'll explore grounding techniques—practices designed to keep you anchored, even when life feels like it's pulling you in every direction. Together, we'll deepen this connection and discover new ways to find steadiness, no matter what comes your way.

5

FIND YOUR ANCHOR: GROUNDING TECHNIQUES

WHAT DOES it mean to feel steady in your body? After trauma, that steadiness can feel unfamiliar—like trying to walk on a floor that keeps shifting beneath you. You already know how trauma traps the nervous system in survival mode, flipping between hyper-alertness and complete shutdown. It's draining, and it pulls you out of the present moment, leaving your mind stuck bracing for a threat that's no longer there.

Grounding techniques work like a stabilizer, easing the overwhelm and drawing you back into the present moment. It's not about forcing calm when it feels out of reach or rewriting the patterns trauma left behind. Instead, it's about reconnecting with what's happening *right now*, offering your body a way to tap into the steadying rhythm of the present.

Let's jump in and explore how to turn this concept into a lifesaver when life feels anything but steady.

Finding Your Footing With Grounding: Exercises

Some exercises are quick and subtle—easy to work into the chaos of a busy day—while others invite you to slow down and connect more

FIND YOUR ANCHOR: GROUNDING TECHNIQUES 63

deeply. The goal is to give yourself a moment to shift out of overwhelm and back into something steadier. Let's dive into a few ways to make grounding work for you.

Exercise 15: Sole Connection

You know that moment when you finally kick off your shoes after a long day and feel the cool floor beneath your feet? That's the perfect opportunity to pause and reconnect with yourself. This exercise is all about noticing the ground beneath you—its textures, its steady support—and letting that awareness bring you back to the present.

1. Stand barefoot on a surface that feels comfortable, such as hardwood, grass, or carpet.
2. Let your feet rest naturally and begin to shift your weight slowly from your heels to your toes.
3. Notice the sensations under your feet—the texture, temperature, and firmness.
4. Focus on the feeling of the ground supporting you as you shift your weight back and forth. Notice the stability under your feet and how it holds you without effort.
5. Continue for 1–2 minutes, paying attention to any changes in how your body feels.

Using the provided drawing below, mark the sensations you noticed during the exercise:

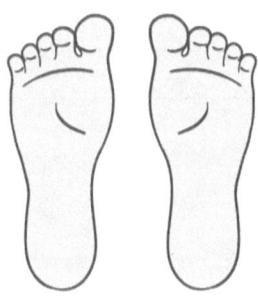

- **lines** for areas of pressure
- **dots** for warmth or coolness
- **colors** to represent grounded or connected regions (e.g., blue for coolness, red for warmth)

Exercise 16: Grounding With an Anchoring Statement

When your brain feels like it is running in five directions at once, an anchoring statement can bring you back to the present. It's a quick way to remind yourself where you are, what's around you, and that you're okay.

1. Start with the basics. Say your name, where you are, and what time it is. No overthinking—just the facts. "I'm Jamie. I'm 27, sitting on my couch. It's Wednesday at 6:42 p.m."
2. Take in your surroundings. What's around you? What small details stand out? "The lamp next to me is warm and glowing. My sweater is soft. I can hear cars outside."
3. Say what's next. What are you about to do? Even something tiny counts. "I'm going to take a deep breath, sip my tea, and text my friend back."

Your turn:

- Write your full anchoring statement here:

_____
_____
_____

Exercise 17: Breathe and Press

Imagine sitting at your desk, your mind swirling with thoughts about everything you need to do. Or maybe you're standing in your kitchen after a long day, feeling like the world is still spinning too fast. This simple exercise is here for moments like these—a grounding practice that pairs steady pressure with deep breathing to help you hit pause and find your center.

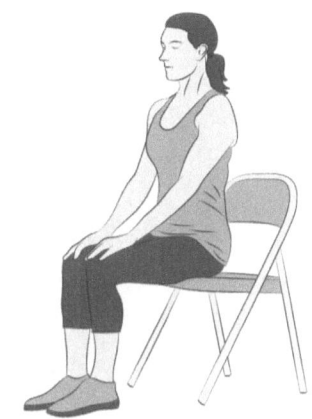

1. Sit or stand in a comfortable position.
2. Place your hands on your thighs or a flat surface in front of you.
3. Inhale deeply through your nose, pressing your palms firmly into the surface.
4. Hold the pressure for a moment, then exhale slowly through your mouth as you release.
5. Repeat this motion 3–5 times, noticing how the physical action calms your mind and steadies your body.

After completing all repetitions, rest your palms flat on the surface and take a moment to observe:

- How does your body feel now? What do you notice about your posture, balance, or sense of stability?

_____
_____
_____

Exercise 18: Nature Walk With Intention

Nature isn't just a backdrop—it's like a reset button for your nervous system. Research has found that spending at least 120 minutes a week in natural environments is linked to better health and well-being (White et al., 2019). Just two hours! That's less time than most of us spend scrolling through social media in a day.

Walking in nature becomes even more grounding when you engage your senses one at a time.

Try this simple practice to help reconnect with the world around you:

1. Take a walk in a natural setting—a park, forest, beach, or garden.
2. As you walk, focus on one sensory experience at a time:
   - Start with sight: Notice the colors, shapes, and light around you.
   - Shift to sound: Listen to birdsong, rustling leaves, or distant waves.
   - Move to touch: Feel the air on your skin, the texture of leaves, or the coolness of a stone in your hand.
3. Let each step become an act of connection, tethering you to the present through the natural world.

After your walk, pause and consider:

- What did you notice that you hadn't before?

_____
_____
_____

- Were there moments when your senses pulled you into a deeper awareness?

These grounding exercises are like the roots of a tree, steadying you in the moment and helping you reconnect with the present. But what happens when the tension you're feeling isn't just about the here and now? When it's tied to deeper emotions or past experiences that linger and weigh on you? That's where a more targeted approach, like EFT tapping, can help.

EFT Tapping: Releasing Trauma One Tap at a Time

Scrolling through TikTok one day, I came across a video that perfectly captured the essence of EFT tapping, short for Emotional Freedom Technique. The creator shared their story of growing up with a scarcity mindset around money. Seeing others struggle financially left an emotional imprint that shaped their own beliefs. Over time, those beliefs held them back from achieving their goals. But through EFT tapping, they started breaking free from those deeply ingrained patterns, working through emotional blocks tied to past experiences and rewiring their thought processes to open up new possibilities.

So, what exactly is EFT tapping, and how does it work? At its core, it's a mind-body technique that blends gentle tapping on acupressure points with focused attention on a thought, memory, or emotion. These points align with energy pathways used in acupuncture, but instead of needles, you use your fingertips to stimulate them. This process helps calm your nervous system, reduce stress, and release emotional tension stored in your body (Rush & Leonard, 2019), while also creating space for a shift in perspective that loosens the hold of limiting beliefs and unhelpful thought patterns.

This is how it works: You're tapping lightly on specific points—like the side of your hand or your collarbone—while focusing on something that's weighing you down. Maybe it's an old memory, a nagging belief, or just a feeling you can't shake. Instead of trying to force yourself into "thinking positive," EFT tapping works directly with your body to help shift those emotions.

We have explored how unresolved emotions don't just fade away. They linger, shaping the way you react to certain situations without you even realizing it. This is especially true with trauma, where emotionally charged memories form neural pathways that reinforce old patterns. EFT tapping helps interrupt those patterns. By stimulating acupressure points while recalling a difficult memory, you send calming signals to your brain—specifically to the amygdala and hippocampus, the areas responsible for processing fear and stress (König et al., 2019).

The best way to understand EFT tapping, though, is to experience it for yourself. Let's break it down into five simple steps so you can try it firsthand.

Exercise 19: EFT Tapping

1. Start by choosing a specific issue to address. Maybe it's the knot of anxiety before a big meeting, or the lingering sadness of an unresolved argument. Get as specific as possible and write it down:
    - The issue I am addressing is _____ and the emotion that I'm focusing on is _____.
2. Rate how strongly you're experiencing the issue or emotion on a scale of 0–10, with 10 being the most intense and 0 being no intensity at all. This will help you track your progress through the exercise.
    - Circle your starting intensity: 0 1 2 3 4 5 6 7 8 9 10
    - Take a moment to notice where you feel the intensity in your body. Is it in your chest, your stomach, or

somewhere else?

_____

3. Before tapping, create a simple phrase that acknowledges your issue and expresses self-acceptance, as this will help center your focus during the sequence. A common setup phrase is: "Even though I have this [issue], I deeply and completely accept myself." You can also personalize it to fit your specific situation. For example:
   - "Even though I feel anxious about that conversation, I deeply and completely accept myself."
   - "Even though I'm frustrated about the argument, I accept and support myself."
     - Now it's your turn, write your setup phrase here:
     _____

4. Now that you've created your setup phrase, it's time to begin tapping.
   - Start by gently tapping the **side of your hand** (known as the "karate chop" point) while repeating your setup phrase three times. This step helps establish your focus and prepares your body and mind for the sequence.
   - Next, move through the tapping points listed below, tapping each one about seven times. As you tap, repeat a short reminder phrase that reflects your setup, such as "this anxiety in my stomach" or "this frustration in my neck."
     - **Eyebrow (EB):** inside edge of the eyebrow.
     - **Side of the eye (SE):** near the temple.
     - **Under the eye (UE):** on the cheekbone.
     - **Under the nose (UN):** between the nose and upper lip.
     - **Chin (Ch):** between the lower lip and chin.
     - **Collarbone (CB):** just below the collarbone.
     - **Under the arm (UA):** about four inches below the armpit.

- **Top of the head (TH):** center of the crown.
    - Repeat the sequence two or three times, moving through the points in order.

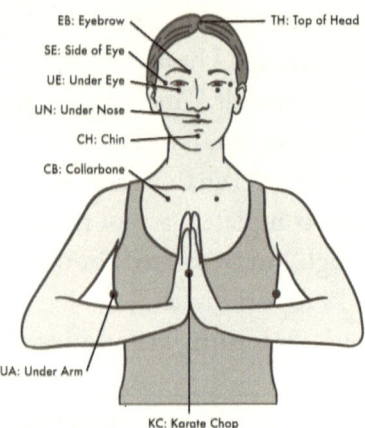

After completing the tapping sequence, take a moment to reassess the intensity of your issue:

- Circle your ending intensity: 0 1 2 3 4 5 6 7 8 9 10

Pause and check in with yourself:

- How did the intensity change for you? What did you notice?

_____
_____
_____

- What physical or emotional shifts did you feel in your body?

_____

_____

_____

Did a different emotion come up after completing the sequence? If so, you can now repeat the tapping process while focusing on this new emotion. Some memories hold multiple emotional layers, and tapping can help you work through them one at a time.

If you find that this technique isn't producing noticeable results, try getting more specific. Instead of focusing on a general event or feeling, hone in on a particular detail that stands out—such as the look on someone's face, a specific phrase that was said, or a moment that triggered a strong emotional response. Often, it's the small, specific details that hold the most emotional charge.

EFT tapping is powerful because it helps us connect inward, addressing the blocks we carry within ourselves. But sometimes, grounding and balance aren't just about what's happening inside us—they're also about how we navigate the world around us. Setting boundaries, whether with people, situations, or even your own habits, is another way to create clarity and safety in your life.

Why Boundaries Matter: Protecting Your Peace

Think of boundaries as an extension of grounding. If grounding helps you find your footing, boundaries are what help you keep it. They give you the freedom to say, "This is enough for me today," or, "I need to step back," without shutting yourself off completely. Instead of walls, think of them as doors you can open or close depending on what feels safe and supportive.

For many of us, setting boundaries doesn't come naturally—especially if you've spent years prioritizing others or identifying as a "people pleaser." At first, it might feel heavy, like you're letting someone down or being selfish. But boundaries aren't selfish. They're acts of self-respect. They're a way of saying, "I matter, too."

And while some boundaries are easy to set, others can feel uncomfortable but ultimately bring the most clarity and peace.

A colleague once shared how setting a boundary at work transformed her life. She always said yes—taking on extra projects, late-night emails, and meetings that weren't hers. The stress showed up in tension headaches, restless nights, and Sunday night anxiety. On Friday at 6 p.m., when her boss handed her another project, she took a deep breath and said, "I'd be happy to help, but I need more time to do it right." To her surprise, her boss apologized and reassessed workloads. At first, she felt guilty, but soon she realized she hadn't let others down—she'd only been letting herself down. "I didn't stop being a team player," she said. "I just started respecting my own boundaries."

Your body often knows when a boundary is needed before your mind does. That tightening in your chest when someone asks for more than you can give, the sinking feeling when you agree to something you don't want to do, or that lingering sense of disappointment within yourself when you ignore what you need—these aren't weaknesses. They're your body's way of saying, "This doesn't feel right." Listening to those signals is the first step toward setting boundaries that protect your peace.

So, let's dive into some practical ways to do that—ones that feel natural, honor your body, respect your limits, and create space for what truly supports you.

Drawing the Line By Setting Boundaries: Techniques

Boundaries are deeply personal, shaped by your experiences, needs, and limits. Learning to set them takes practice and intention. It's not about saying "no" to everything, but about learning when to say "yes" to yourself. Grounding techniques and somatic awareness provide a powerful foundation for this work, helping you notice what your body needs and how to honor it.

Exercise 20: Toward and Away

Ever felt someone standing a little *too* close in line and wanted to casually step back? That's your body's way of saying, "Nope, this is my bubble." This exercise helps you fine-tune that awareness. Whether you're working with a partner or just imagining someone approaching, you'll learn to notice those "stop right there" signals your body sends. It's like getting a built-in radar for your personal space—handy for everything from crowded elevators to tricky conversations.

You can do this solo or with a partner:

- **With a partner**: They'll be the one approaching, and you'll communicate when they should stop.
  - **A quick note:** Partner here just means another person—like a friend. A romantic partner might not be the best fit, as you may already feel at ease with them.
- **Alone**: Visualize someone stepping closer in your mind and notice how your body reacts.

Let's try it:

1. Stand in a clear space or sit in a sturdy chair where you feel at ease.
2. If you're with a partner, ask them to start a few steps away and approach slowly. If you're solo, picture someone in your mind taking steps toward you.
3. Say "stop" when you feel the need. Notice how your body reacts in that moment—do your shoulders tense, does your breath change, or do you feel a pull to move back?
4. Try the exercise again with small changes:
   - Adjust the speed of the approach.

- Imagine or have your partner approach from different angles.
- Observe how these variations shift your comfort level.

Use the prompts below to capture what you noticed during the exercise:

- When I said stop, I felt _____ in my body.
- I knew it was the right distance because:

_____
_____
_____

- How did your reaction change when the person approached from a different angle or at a different speed? Did you feel more or less comfortable? Did you want to say "stop" sooner or later?

_____
_____
_____

- Lastly, imagine using this in real life. For example, if someone gets too close during a conversation, what might it feel like to politely assert your boundary?

_____
_____
_____

Exercise 21: Like It/Don't Like It

We all have opinions about what feels right in relationships, but naming them can feel like guessing what's in a mystery box. This exercise is your chance to sort out the "yes, please" from the "not a chance." By creating a simple scale—either by moving around the room or sketching it out—you'll get a clear view of your preferences. Plus, you might stumble on a pattern you didn't realize was there.

Let's break it down:

1. Start by creating your scale.
    - If you want to move physically, choose one side of the room as "I love it" and the opposite as "I dislike it."
    - If using paper feels more your style, draw a line with one end marked "I love it" and the other "I dislike it."
2. Use the statements below to explore your preferences. Think about where you'd place yourself on the scale for each one:

- I feel more comfortable when someone asks before stepping in to help.
- I prefer to process my emotions alone before talking.
- I like resolving conflict immediately rather than waiting.
- I feel supported when someone listens without giving advice.
- Try writing two of your own statements to explore. These could be situations that come up often in your relationships or areas where you feel unsure about your preferences:

3. As you go through the exercise, notice your body's reactions to each statement. Do you feel a sense of ease or tension as you make your choices? These physical signals can give you clues about your boundaries and preferences.

To help solidify what you've learned, reflect on these questions:

- When I think about my responses above, one pattern I see is:

- I feel grounded and supported when:

- One preference I didn't realize I had until now is:

Exercise 22: Exploring Boundaries With Hands

Your hands are like boundary experts. In this exercise, you'll use them to map out your personal space—exploring what feels safe, comfortable, or in need of a boundary. Imagine a person or situation, and let your hands do the talking. It's simple, intuitive, and a little like waving a magic wand to say, "Here's where I draw the line." By the end, you'll know exactly how to hold your space with confidence—and maybe even a little flair.

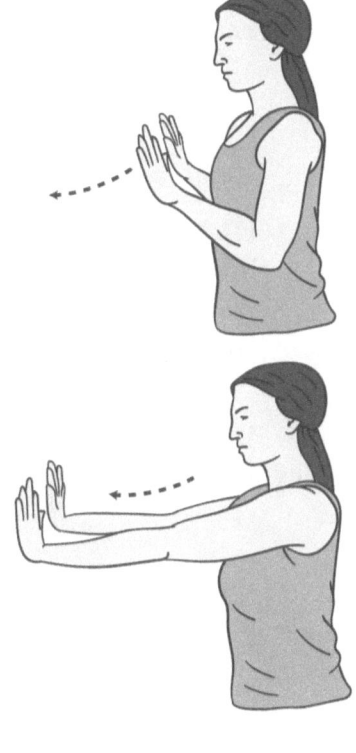

1. Find a spot where you can move your arms freely. Stand or sit somewhere you feel relaxed, letting your shoulders drop, and your hands rest naturally at your sides.
2. Start moving your hands, palms facing outward. Slowly bring them closer to your body, then push them farther away. Notice how the distance feels: Does closer make you feel protected or crowded? Does further feel freeing or disconnected? Pause when you find a sweet spot that feels just right.
3. If it helps, think about someone specific or a situation you've been in recently. Picture them standing in front of you and use your hands to map out how far or close you'd want them to be. If imagining feels tricky, grab a stand-in object—a pillow, chair, or whatever's nearby—and experiment with how your boundary shifts.
4. Play around with hand positions—palms in, palms out, one hand closer than the other. How do these subtle changes affect your sense of comfort? There's no wrong

way to do this. The goal is to notice what feels protective, supportive, or empowering for you.

As you worked through this, you might have noticed that some movements felt calming, while others made you feel stronger or more in control. Let's take it a step further: Connect a physical gesture with an emotion that helps you hold your boundaries.

For example:

- Palms out might feel like calm, giving you space to breathe.
- A wide, open stance could feel like confidence, letting you own your space.

Now, think about the emotions that matter most when setting boundaries. Which hand positions match those feelings?

- _____
- _____
- _____
- _____

Each of these techniques is a chance to connect your body's signals with your personal boundaries, helping you tune into what feels right for you. Boundaries aren't just about managing relationships—they're about understanding yourself on a deeper level. As you practice, you might notice subtle but powerful changes: a confidence that comes from honoring your limits and the ability to hold space for your needs without second-guessing yourself.

Boundaries don't exist in isolation—they're part of a bigger picture. They work hand in hand with grounding practices to help you feel steady, clear, and present in your day-to-day life. Imagine coming home after a long, draining day—your body feels tense, your mind is scattered, and a friend calls to vent about their problems. Instead of automatically saying yes, grounding helps you check in with yourself first. You take a deep breath, feel your feet on the floor, and notice your exhaustion. With this awareness, you set a boundary: *"I want to be there for you, but I need to rest first. Can we talk tomorrow?"* In that moment, grounding helps you tune in, and boundaries help you follow through.

There's no perfect way to do this—it's a practice, not a personality trait you either have or don't. Some days, you'll hold your boundaries like a Zen master. Other days, you'll let one slide and only realize it later when you're stuck in a conversation you didn't have the energy for. But each time you pause, center yourself, or say no when it matters, you're strengthening something important: Trust in yourself. Not just the belief that you *can* navigate life's chaos, but the quiet knowing that you *deserve* to do it in a way that works for you.

From here, it's not just about staying steady—it's about leveling up. How do you not just hold your ground but tap into your body's natural strengths to move through life with more ease and confidence? In the next part of this journey, we're going to dive into somatic therapy practices, kicking things off with breathwork.

6

BREATHE IN, HEAL OUT: THE POWER OF BREATHWORK

BREATHING DOESN'T USUALLY MAKE headlines, but I think it should. It's the one thing you've been doing since the moment you were born. Breathing is a reflex for all of us—it happens without much thought. But have you ever considered that your breath might hold more potential than simply keeping you alive?

Ancient cultures certainly thought so. Indian yogis practiced *pranayama*, a form of breath control, not just as a breathing exercise but to control energy and restore balance (Egberts, 2023). Across Asia, monks used breath like a tuning fork, sharpening focus and creating stillness in meditation. Indigenous groups wove breath into rituals, treating it as a bridge between the physical and the spiritual. Long before science caught up, people understood that breath was more than just air—it was influence.

Fast-forward to today, and research backs what these traditions have known for centuries. A study in the *Cyprus Journal of Medical Sciences* found that controlled breathing reduces cortisol levels, the hormone responsible for stress (Örün et al., 2021). In other words, the way you breathe directly impacts whether your nervous system is on high alert or in rest-and-repair mode.

This is because breath isn't just a reaction—it's a messenger.

Shallow, rapid breathing tells your body there's danger, triggering stress responses even if there's no real threat. Slow, deep breaths send the opposite signal, telling your system it's safe to relax, reset, and restore. It's one of the few functions that are both automatic and under your control, which makes it an effective tool for shifting your state in real time.

If this sounds too easy to be effective, that's exactly what makes it so powerful. In a world with so many solutions to stress, your breath is one of the simplest and most accessible tools you have. When used with intention, it becomes more than just survival—it becomes a guide, a reset button, a direct line to a calmer, clearer you.

And yet, most of us don't think about it until we're already off balance—tight shoulders, restless mind, that wired-but-exhausted feeling. Those are signals, and breathwork offers a way to respond. Let's explore the benefits and see how small shifts in your breath can create big changes.

Benefits of Breathwork

You know that moment when you finally sit down after a long day, let out a deep sigh, and realize just how much tension you've been holding? That's your body's way of reminding you it's been carrying more than it should.

I had one of those days not long ago—the kind that leaves you running on fumes before you even realize it. My six-month-old wouldn't stop crying, my toddler was tugging at my shirt with toy after toy, and the house looked like a tornado had swept through it. By the time I caved and took the bubbles from my toddler's hand, I was running on empty. My plan? Blow enough bubbles to distract her so I could get a minute of quiet. But as I sat down and took a deep breath in to blow, something unexpected happened.

That long, slow exhale felt... different. By the third breath, I noticed a calm creeping in. My shoulders dropped, my mind cleared, and it was as if someone had flipped a switch inside me. What were the chances? I thought I was just blowing bubbles to entertain my toddler, but somehow, I was grounding myself in the process.

Later, I realized those deep breaths were activating my parasympathetic nervous system—the part of the body that tells everything to relax, to settle. Turns out, it wasn't just a distraction for my kid; it was exactly what I needed, too.

Beyond that, research confirms that this practice positively impacts both your body and your brain:

- **Lifts your mood:** Research shows that breath-focused practices can ease symptoms of depression and boost emotional resilience, helping you feel more balanced (Zaccaro et al., 2018).
- **Sharpens focus:** Deep, deliberate breaths send more oxygen to your brain, enhancing clarity and helping you stay alert without feeling drained (Brown & Gerbarg, 2005).
- **Improves sleep:** A few minutes of rhythmic breathing before bed can lower cortisol levels, setting the stage for a more restful night (Lee et al., 2021).

There's another perk: self-compassion. I don't know about you, but most of us are way harder on ourselves than we are on anyone else. Breathwork has this sneaky way of softening that inner voice. As you connect with your body and pay attention to what it needs, you start to treat yourself with the same care and kindness you'd offer a friend. And honestly, don't we all need a little more of that?

In a minute, we're going to dive into some exercises, and it is important to remember that there's no one-size-fits-all approach to breathwork, so you'll get to try a few exercises to see what resonates with you. Maybe you'll find one that calms you down after a stressful day, or another that helps you recharge when your energy feels low.

So, let's keep this momentum going. You've learned how powerful your breath can be—now it's time to experience it for yourself.

Harnessing the Power of Breath: Exercises

Now that we've explored how your breath can support your body and mind, let's get practical.

Exercise 23: Diaphragmatic Breathing

This one's the bread and butter of somatic breathwork. It helps you breathe deeply and efficiently, grounding you when stress takes over —like when you're feeling jittery before hosting a family gathering or trying to unwind after an adrenaline-filled day.

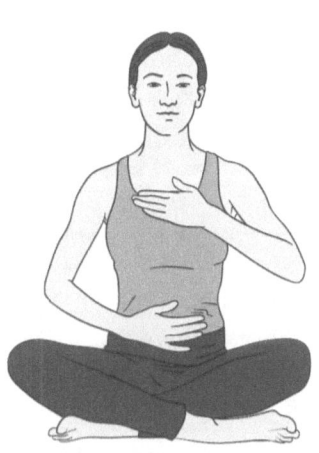

1. Find a spot where you can relax. Sit upright in a chair or lie down with your back supported.
2. Place one hand on your chest and the other on your belly.
3. Inhale deeply through your nose. Feel your belly rise under your hand, while your chest stays as still as possible.
4. Exhale slowly through your mouth, letting your belly fall.
5. Repeat for 5–10 minutes, focusing on the gentle rhythm of your breath.

As you settle into the flow, take a moment to check in with yourself:

- How do you feel emotionally before and after practicing diaphragmatic breathing? Do you notice any shifts in mood, stress levels, or energy?

- As you breathe deeply into your diaphragm, what do you notice happening in your body? Do you feel a sense of expansion, relaxation, or resistance?

This technique is especially helpful when you're trying to transition from "go-go-go" mode into restful sleep or when you need a moment of calm in the middle of a chaotic day.

Exercise 24: Somatic Sighing

Sometimes, a good sigh is all you need. This technique works wonders when you're stuck in a long traffic jam or processing an emotionally charged conversation.

1. Sit comfortably, resting your hands on your lap.
2. Take a deep breath in through your nose, filling your lungs completely.
3. Exhale with an audible sigh. Let it be long and drawn out —don't hold back.
4. Repeat 5–10 times, and notice how each sigh feels lighter than the last.

After a few rounds, ask yourself:

- On a scale from 1 to 10, how tense did you feel before starting?

BREATHE IN, HEAL OUT: THE POWER OF BREATHWORK

- How would you rate your tension now?

_____
_____
_____

It might feel a bit unfamiliar at first, but trust me—your body knows what to do with a good, honest sigh.

Exercise 25: Somatic Breath Counting

When your thoughts are racing—like when you're trying to focus in a loud café or calm your nerves before hitting "send" on an important email—this exercise helps you pause and ground yourself.

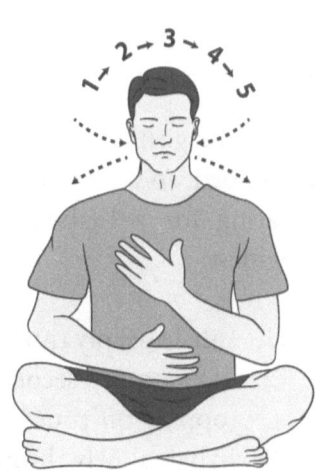

1. Sit with your back straight, hands resting on your knees.
2. Close your eyes and take a slow breath in through your nose.
3. As you exhale, silently count "one."
4. Repeat with each exhale, counting up to 10. Then start back at one.
5. Practice for 5–10 minutes, letting the counting guide your focus.

Check-in with yourself:

- Describe any physical sensations you experienced during the practice (e.g., tension, relaxation, warmth, tingling).

___

- Did you notice any patterns while counting (such as losing track, feeling distracted, or becoming restless)? What might this tell you about your current state of mind?

___

If you catch your mind wandering, gently bring it back to the count.

Exercise 26: The Double Inhale Method

Feeling sluggish? This technique is perfect when you've just rolled out of bed and need to kickstart your morning, or when you're preparing for a high-energy workout but can't quite shake the grogginess.

1. Inhale deeply through your nose.
2. Take a quick second inhale right after, as if you're topping off your lungs.
3. Exhale slowly through your mouth, emptying your lungs completely.
4. Repeat for 1–2 minutes, noticing how your energy shifts.

As you finish, notice the difference in your alertness:

- How alert do you feel now compared to before?

_____
_____
_____

- Did your body feel more energized, or did you notice any tension release?

_____
_____
_____

This exercise can be a lifesaver for those mid-afternoon slumps—or any time you need a quick pick-me-up.

Exercise 27: Bilateral Stimulation

This exercise is ideal when you're feeling out of sync—like after a long day of decision-making or when you're recovering from an intense conversation that left you emotionally drained.

1. Sit upright in a comfortable position.
2. Inhale deeply through your nose.
3. As you exhale, snap your fingers on your left hand, then your right, followed by a clap.
4. Repeat this pattern for 1–2 minutes, letting the sounds and movements sync with your breath.

After you open your eyes, you can ask yourself:

- How would you describe your overall state after finishing the exercise?

- How has this exercise shifted your awareness or focus?

This one can feel a little playful—lean into it! Sometimes, shaking up the routine is exactly what your body needs.

As you tried these exercises, what stood out to you? Did one feel easier or more natural than the others? Maybe one challenged you in a way that made you pause and think. Take a moment to jot down your thoughts or simply sit with them. These insights will help you deepen your practice and discover what works best for you.

Breathwork is as much about exploration as it is about the breath itself. Each exercise is an invitation to connect with yourself on a deeper level, to notice what your body is telling you, and to respond with care and intention. So, which one will you try again first?

When you're ready, let's move forward and explore ways to weave these practices into your daily routine.

Incorporating Breathwork Into Your Daily Life

By now, you've seen what breathwork can do, and the best part? It doesn't need to be a grand production. You don't have to block off hours or hunt for the perfect setting. Breathwork is more like a subtle thread you can weave into your day—it's not the centerpiece, but it quietly holds everything together.

So, how do you fit it into an already packed day? Let's break it down with three simple exercises you can weave into your day.

Exercise 28: The Traffic Light Breath

When you're stopped at a red light, instead of letting frustration bubble up, turn it into a moment of grounding.

1. Rest one hand on your chest and the other on your belly.
2. Inhale deeply through your nose, feeling both hands rise with your breath.
3. Pause briefly at the top, then exhale slowly through your mouth, noticing your hands fall.
4. Repeat until the light turns green, using the rhythm of your breath to center yourself.

Try it next time you're stuck in traffic and notice how your body shifts—does the frustration ease, even just a little?

Exercise 29: The Elevator Breather

Whether you're riding an elevator or waiting for one, this exercise turns a small pause into a moment of calm.

1. Stand with your hands relaxed at your sides and your feet slightly apart.
2. Breathe in deeply as the elevator begins to move up or down, but only for a few seconds—don't hold your breath for the entire ride.
3. Pause briefly at a natural point in your breath when the elevator stops at a floor.
4. Exhale slowly as the elevator's doors open.
5. Repeat for as many floors as you need, allowing your breath to flow naturally and comfortably with the movement of the elevator.

How does it feel to sync your breath with something external?

Notice if the rhythm leaves you feeling steadier by the time you step out.

The more these practices become part of your routine, the more you'll notice a shift in your breathing and in the way you connect with your body. Breathwork turns into your personal tuning mechanism, clearing out the static so you can catch your body's quiet messages. Every mindful breath becomes a clever reminder: "I'm listening."

Now that you've started tuning in through breathwork, we're ready to build on that foundation. In the next chapter, Build Resilience: Resourcing and Sequencing, we'll dive into practical tools that help you harness both your internal and external resources.

Make a Difference with Your Review

"Healing yourself is connected with healing others."

— YOKO ONO

Somewhere out there, there's someone just like you—curious about somatic therapy, searching for a way to feel better in their own skin, hoping for a guide to help them reconnect with their body. Maybe they're scrolling through books, unsure which one will actually help. That's where *you* come in.

Most people choose books based on reviews. Your words could be the reason someone decides to take that first step toward healing. It costs nothing, takes less than a minute, but could change everything for someone else.

Your review could help...
- ...one more person discover the power of somatic therapy.
- ...one more nervous system find balance.
- ...one more body release tension and find ease.
- ...one more person realize they are not alone in their journey.

To make a difference, simply scan the QR code and leave a review: https://www.amazon.com/review/review-your-purchases/?asin=1764076109

If you love helping others, you're my kind of person. Thank you from the bottom of my heart!

— Sarrah Kaye

7

BUILD RESILIENCE: RESOURCING AND SEQUENCING

Now, we're diving into the key practices that define somatic therapy, starting with Somatic Experiencing® (SE). Originally developed by Dr. Peter A. Levine, SE is a trauma-healing method that works directly with the nervous system (*SE 101*, n.d.). Think about it like when a movie freezes right before the resolution—you're stuck in the intensity, unable to move forward. SE helps "press play" again, allowing the body to finish its natural protective responses and finally find relief. Instead of dragging you through painful memories, it taps into the body's natural ability to heal, offering a gentler, more biologically attuned way to recover from trauma.

If you think back to earlier chapters, we explored how trauma affects the body and leaves the autonomic nervous system (ANS) stuck in fight, flight, or freeze mode. Remember those brain regions we talked about—the amygdala, our built-in threat detector, and the prefrontal cortex, which handles decision-making and keeps emotions in check? Trauma throws those areas off balance. SE steps in here, using body-focused techniques to gently recalibrate the nervous system, restoring that lost communication between your brain and body so they can team up again (*SE 101*, n.d.).

Now, you might be wondering: How does SE actually do this? It uses guiding principles that mirror how your nervous system naturally heals when it's given the right tools. Each of these plays a critical role in helping your body shift from survival mode back to balance. Here's a sneak peek:

- **Titration** is about approaching challenging memories or sensations in small doses—like adding dye drop by drop to a glass of water instead of pouring it all in at once. This gentle pacing helps prevent overwhelm, so your nervous system can process gradually.
- **Pendulation** leverages the body's natural swing between activation and calm. You allow yourself to feel a bit of distress, and then you deliberately switch to moments of ease or neutral sensations, moving back and forth between the two. Over time, this back-and-forth builds resilience and self-regulation.
- **Resourcing** means tapping into anything that fosters a sense of safety, comfort, or strength, whether it's a soothing memory, a supportive person, or even a grounded feeling in your own body. It's generally used as an anchor during pendulation and titration exercises, giving you a safe place to return to if things start to feel overwhelming.
- **Tracking** is a term we explored in chapter 4. It's the practice of noticing and mapping your bodily sensations without judgment. This skill builds a foundation for deeper somatic work, making it easier to recognize patterns, release tension, and move toward regulation.
- **Sequencing** is all about processing emotions in the right order, so you're not hit with everything all at once. Think of it like following a recipe—each step builds on the one before, helping you stay steady and avoid feeling overwhelmed. We'll dive into sequencing a bit later in this chapter, but for now, just know it's a key skill for managing emotional flow.

- **SIBAM (Sensation, Image, Behavior, Affect, and Meaning)** isn't a technique but a framework that helps you understand your experience when practicing tracking, pendulation, and titration. It helps connect sensations, thoughts, emotions, and actions, making it easier to process what's stuck. Say your chest tightens, your breath shortens (sensation), and a memory surfaces of being put on the spot in a meeting (image). That discomfort makes you shrink back and avoid speaking up (behavior), while frustration or shame lingers (affect), reinforcing the belief that you're not capable or will be judged if you don't have the perfect response (meaning). SIBAM helps you recognize these patterns so you can work through them instead of staying stuck.

All these principles work together to help your body complete the protective responses it never got to finish, releasing stored tension bit by bit. While the purpose of somatic awareness is to recognize those stuck sensations, what makes SE different is its focus on active body-based exercises. You don't have to relive every painful detail of your past; rather, you learn to listen to what your body is saying now, intervene with supportive resources, and let your system unwind at a pace it can handle.

We'll explore these terms and concepts more as we move forward, seeing how they play out in the practice of SE and contribute to healing.

Benefits of Somatic Experiencing®

Beyond the core principles we just explored, you might be wondering, "What can I actually *gain* from this approach?" Well, let's talk results for a second. In a randomized controlled study, SE had some impressive outcomes. Participants with PTSD saw their symptom severity drop significantly—from an average score of 68.4 to 36.3 on the Clinician-Administered PTSD Scale (CAPS)—indicating a major improvement (Brom et al., 2017). Depression symptoms also fell by over 30%, showing that SE doesn't just address emotional distress but also helps restore overall well-being. Here's a glimpse of what it can offer:

- less emotional overload, so stress doesn't hit like a tidal wave, making it easier to process emotions without feeling consumed by them (Brom et al., 2017).
- sharper focus and a clearer mind by helping your nervous system find balance, so you're not stuck in a fog of stress and overthinking (Cellarius, 2023).
- better sleep and more energy because when your body isn't stuck in survival mode, you get to rest and recharge (Brom et al., 2017).
- a sense of empowerment and hope as you move past old patterns, feel lighter, and realize you're not just surviving—you're moving forward (Cellarius, 2023).

This is just a snapshot of the potential benefits. As you continue your journey, you may discover even more ways in which it enriches your life. As we continue, we'll explore how these changes happen on a practical level and how you can begin weaving somatic practices into your daily life.

Resourcing: Building Inner Strength and Resilience

Think of resourcing as your emotional life jacket—it won't stop the waves from crashing, but it'll keep you afloat long enough to find steadier ground. In Somatic Experiencing®, resourcing is about finding those small, steady moments that help you feel supported, especially when navigating heavier somatic practices like titration or pendulation. It's not about erasing discomfort but creating space to remind your body, "Hey, I've got this." These resources can be anything positive and embodied that helps you reconnect—like a comforting memory or a soothing sensation. They're your nervous system's way of accessing a felt sense of safety, support, and nourishment that you can build and return to, moment by moment (Lozovyi, 2022).

Why is it so important? Well, diving into big feelings without a safety net can feel like hiking a steep trail without the right gear—overwhelming and unsteady. Resourcing steps in when your nervous system is stuck in overdrive, giving it a gentle nudge toward calm.

Your resources might be anything that feels comforting, grounding, or steady. A memory of sipping hot chocolate on a snowy day, the rhythm of your favorite song, or even the feel of your favorite hoodie's soft fabric against your skin. These are your tools to remind your body that safety is possible, even in the middle of chaos.

Let's paint a picture: You're sitting at your desk, trying to focus, when an email pops up. It's not just any email—it's *that* email from *that* person. Suddenly, your stomach drops, your chest tightens, and your thoughts spiral into every worst-case scenario. What's wild is that this email isn't the real issue—it's the way it hit an old nerve, stirring up a memory or feeling you thought was buried. Cue the body's overreaction.

Now, imagine that instead of spiraling, you pause. You think about a moment that feels the opposite of what you're experiencing right now. Maybe it's the memory of lying on your couch, a warm blanket wrapped around you, binge-watching your favorite comfort show. Or the feeling of standing outside on a crisp fall day, with leaves crunching under your boots. As you let your mind rest on that moment, your shoulders start to ease, your breathing slows, and you feel less like a bundle of live wires. That's resourcing: creating a pocket of calm to remind your body that it doesn't have to stay in fight, flight or freeze mode forever.

The magic of resourcing isn't that it fixes everything—it doesn't need to. It just helps you create a bubble of safety to catch your breath and find your footing when things feel overwhelming. And the more you practice, the better you'll get at spotting those small but mighty moments of steadiness, even when life feels chaotic.

Up next, we'll dive into some practical exercises to help you uncover and nurture your own unique resources.

Tools to Find Stability: Resourcing Exercises

Resourcing works best when you take the time to explore and identify what feels grounding or comforting for you. Not every resource will resonate deeply, and that's okay. The process is about curiosity—trying out different ideas, noticing what works, and building a personalized toolkit for resilience.

Exercise 30: Five-Step Resourcing

Feeling like life's tugging you in too many directions? Or maybe there's a knot of tension in your chest that just won't budge? This exercise is here to guide you toward steadiness by helping you discover and deepen your internal and external resources. It helps you tap into the calm within the chaos, reminding you that even in tough moments, you're not without support.

1. Take a moment to notice what feels calming, supportive, or grounding for you right now. It could be:
   - the steady contact of your feet on the floor
   - a comforting memory, like the sound of rain or a hug from someone you love
   - a small physical sensation, like warmth in your hands or the rhythm of your breath. If nothing comes to mind, no pressure—just stay open to what might feel good in the moment.
2. Once you've found your resource, give it a name or describe it to yourself. Is it warmth in your chest? A peaceful image? A steady breath? Naming it isn't just about words—it's about anchoring the feeling so you can access it more easily later.

- **Pause Here:** If you're journaling, jot down a word or phrase that captures your resource. No overthinking—just go with what feels right. For example:
    - "It feels like a soft glow in my chest."
    - "This reminds me of sitting in my favorite café, sipping a warm drink."
3. Let yourself fully experience the resource you've identified. What details stand out?
    - Notice its location in your body—where do you feel it most?
    - How does it feel? Is it soft, warm, steady, or light?
    - Can you imagine this resource expanding, like a ripple of calm spreading outward?
4. Stay with the resource for a little bit longer. Let it ground you in the present. When your mind wanders (because it will), gently bring your focus back to what feels steady.
    - Let yourself notice what feels good about this resource.
    - If other thoughts pop up, remind yourself, "I can come back to those later—right now, I'm staying here."

Now that you've spent time with your resource, take a moment to explore how it's affected you.

Reflect on it:

- How does your body feel different—does it feel lighter, warmer, or less tense?

_____
_____
_____

- Do you notice any shifts in your thoughts or mood?

_____
_____
_____

Exercise 31: How Can I Resource Myself?

Learning to identify what activates you and discovering ways to resource yourself is a step toward feeling grounded and in control. This exercise helps you map out your triggers and pair them with resources that bring you back to balance, whether you're feeling over-stimulated or disconnected.

1. Start by reflecting on situations, people, or thoughts that push you into one of three states:
   - **hyper-arousal** (feeling anxious, angry, or overwhelmed)
   - **hypo-arousal** (feeling frozen, withdrawn, or hopeless)
   - **optimum zone of arousal** (feeling balanced, calm, and in control)
     - Write them down. Pay attention to how each trigger feels in your body and mind. Does your heart race? Do you shut down?
2. What helps you feel grounded or connected in those moments? It could be deep belly breathing, stepping outside for fresh air, recalling a kind word from someone you trust, or focusing on a grounding object like a photo or a texture.
3. Match each trigger with a resource. For example:
   - **Hyper-arousal trigger:** Loud arguments at work → **Resource:** Engage your senses by tuning into a neutral or calming sound, like the soft tapping of a keyboard or distant chatter.

- **Hypo-arousal trigger:** Feeling frozen by decision-making → **Resource:** Call a supportive friend or hold a grounding object.
- **Optimum zone of arousal trigger:** A presentation at work with a familiar audience (not too overwhelming) → **Resource:** Use a grounding technique, like pressing your feet into the floor or taking a few deep breaths before speaking.

4. Use the chart below to record your triggers, resources, and the steps you take to transition from activation to balance.

Zone	My triggers are…	My resources are…	I get there by…

5. Once you've filled out the chart, take a moment to think about:

- What patterns did you notice in your triggers, and how do you handle them? What patterns do you see in your resources?

_____
_____
_____

This practice helps you build a toolbox of strategies to regulate your nervous system, expanding your capacity to handle stress over time. But the key to making this work in your daily life is using these tools regularly, not just when things go sideways.

Tips for Using Resourcing Techniques

Resourcing works best when it's something you actually use—not just a last-minute scramble when stress hits like a freight train. The trick? Make it a natural part of your day, so when you need it, it's already second nature. Here are some tips:

1. **Pair resources with neutral sensations:** If your chest feels calm, linger there for a second. If sipping your morning coffee feels like a tiny oasis, let that be a resource. The more you link it to neutral or positive sensations, the easier it is to call on when things get rough. Once you find a resource, go to the table and write it down, or jot it in your journal. That way, it's right there whenever you need it.
2. **Involve the senses:** The more senses you bring in, the stronger the resource. Wrap your hands around a warm mug, breathe in its scent, and feel the weight of it in your palms. Listen to a song that makes your shoulders drop an inch. Layering sensations make resourcing more effective—and honestly, more enjoyable.

3. **Notice what works best:** Not every resource will feel like the one, and that's fine. Some things will click, others won't. Pay attention to what genuinely brings a sense of ease and lean into those.

Resourcing is like unlocking your cheat code for life's chaos. The more you tap into it, the less it feels like a forced strategy and the more it becomes a natural part of your day. That leads us to sequencing—a practice that helps you harness your body's responses into a steady, sustainable rhythm, so you're not simply reacting but actively directing your energy.

Sequencing: Mastering the Flow of Sensations

You know how untangling a set of earbuds feels like a mess until you find the starting point? That's kind of what sequencing is for your body. When sensations feel overwhelming or like they're all jumbled together, sequencing gives you a way to sort through them while letting your body take the lead to follow the natural flow of what it wants to show you next.

Now, don't confuse sequencing with titration (taking things in tiny doses) or pendulation (bouncing between discomfort and ease). Sequencing is about noticing how sensations move through your body, like the natural waves of tension and release.

Here's how you can try it out.

Exercise 32: Sequencing

1. Take a minute to check in with your body. What sensation is grabbing your attention the most right now? Maybe it's a tightness in your shoulders or a flutter in your stomach. Start there, and don't worry about the rest for now—one thing at a time.

2. Spend a little time exploring that sensation. Is it sharp or dull? Does it stay in one spot, or is it moving around? Imagine you're a detective, just noticing the details without trying to change anything. When it starts to shift or fade, let it do its thing.
3. Once that first sensation fades into the background, notice what comes up next. Maybe a new area of tension pops up, or you feel a sense of ease creeping in. Let your body decide the order—it knows what to do.
4. Keep following the flow of sensations, one by one, until your body feels like it's ready to rest. There's no rush, no finish line—just let it unfold naturally.

Over time, you'll notice sequencing doesn't just help you in the moment—it actually builds your capacity to handle sensations and emotions in daily life. It's like strengthening your body's "trust muscle," showing it that it doesn't need to hold onto everything all at once.

When life delivers a punch—whether it's a stomach-churning email, an awkward conversation, or a nagging sense of anxiety—you'll have your resources to lean on. These moments are your chance to reconnect and hit the reset button on your nervous system, bringing you back to calm. Over time, resourcing will become second nature, a steady foundation you can rely on as you dive deeper into somatic practices.

Sequencing, on the other hand, is a bit more like handling fire—it's powerful but might be best approached with guidance. When you start releasing trauma, emotions can bubble up unexpectedly. You might cry, tremble, or feel emotions flood in that you weren't prepared for. But these reactions aren't a sign that something is wrong; they're your body's way of processing and letting go of stored energy.

For everyday stress, you can practice it solo by bringing awareness to subtle bodily shifts—for example, tracking how warmth spreads after deep breathing or how a clenched jaw softens over time. However, if you're dealing with deep trauma or overwhelming emotions, a trained somatic therapist can help pace the experience, ensure safety, and prevent you from getting stuck in distressing sensations.

And remember, this isn't about doing it perfectly or mastering every single tool. It's about experimenting, seeing what clicks, and letting your body guide the process. Healing is personal, and the path forward is all about finding what works for *you*, one small, gentle step at a time.

As we move forward, we'll build on these tools, adding techniques for when emotions feel too heavy for what you've learned so far. Next, we'll explore pendulation and titration—practices designed to help you stay grounded and steady, even in the face of life's most intense emotions.

8

HEAL TRAUMA IN SMALL DOSES: PENDULATION AND TITRATION

Let's take a look at how pendulation and titration fit into the bigger picture. These techniques are the driving force of somatic therapy—the secret ingredients that make it work. They help you gently revisit and release stored experiences without feeling overwhelmed, guiding you to lean into sensations bit by bit while keeping one foot firmly planted in safety.

Keep in mind, working with these practices can sometimes stir up strong emotions, especially when difficult memories or trauma-linked sensations surface. The key is to take it slow—there's no need to dive in headfirst; instead, ease in gently, gradually working your way forward. And if it ever feels like too much, don't hesitate to reach out to a somatic therapist who can help guide you through the process safely.

With that in mind, let's explore these tools in more detail, learning how to use them to navigate sensations safely and build resilience.

Pendulation: Shifting Between Comfort and Discomfort

Think of pendulation like a seesaw. It's not about staying stuck at one extreme but learning to move between discomfort and ease at a steady, manageable pace. With pendulation, you don't dive straight into the deep end of distress—you step into it briefly, then shift back to something that feels safe. Remember those resources you explored in the previous chapter? This is where they come in. They're your reminders of safety, the steady ground you return to after stepping into something challenging—like hiking a steep trail where you pause to catch your breath before moving forward.

For example, say you notice that familiar tightness in your chest—the way your body holds onto a painful memory. With pendulation, you'd explore that sensation for a moment and then shift your focus to your resources, like the feel of your feet pressing into the floor or the sound of your breath. This slow, deliberate rhythm helps your body process those tough feelings in manageable waves, while also reassuring it that it's safe to let go.

Here's what that might look like in therapy: Imagine you're revisiting a difficult memory. As you talk, your chest tightens, your shoulders hunch, your breath turns shallow. Your body's way of saying: *This is a lot.* A somatic therapist's job isn't to tell you to power through. Instead, they'll guide you to pause: *Can you notice the texture of the chair under your hands? Can you focus on the sound of my voice?* Shifting your attention to something neutral gives your body a moment to settle, so when you return to the memory, you're not bracing against it but working through it in a way that feels more in control.

Pendulation is about restoring the rhythm that trauma often disrupts—the natural flow between tension and release, contraction and ease. It's about reminding your nervous system, gently and on its own terms, that it's okay to loosen its grip.

And once you've got that rhythm down? You can slow things down even more by breaking overwhelming moments into even smaller, safer steps with titration.

What Is Titration? Moving Slowly Through Trauma

If pendulation is about finding a rhythm, titration is about slowing that rhythm down to small, bite-sized increments. Think of it like adjusting to bright sunlight after stepping out of a dark room—you don't stare straight into it, you ease in, giving your eyes a moment to adjust. The idea is simple: Breaking a big, overwhelming experience into bite-sized pieces makes it something your body can handle without feeling flooded.

Titration builds on the safety and flow you've practiced with pendulation. Instead of just moving between discomfort and calm, it's about staying with one small piece of what feels challenging. You focus on that fragment, let it settle, and then decide if you're ready for more. This keeps things steady, giving your body the time and space it needs to process what might otherwise feel unmanageable.

Let's say you're working through a memory that feels emotionally charged. Rather than diving into the whole thing, you might focus on one detail that feels more accessible—maybe a fleeting sound or a faint sensation connected to it. That's it. You stay with that one piece just long enough to notice how your body responds, then step back to something grounding using your resources, like a comforting memory or the steady weight of your hands on the table. Titration is about finding that balance: staying with just enough to gently nudge your system forward without pushing it too far.

This slower approach not only keeps things manageable but also gives your nervous system time to integrate what it's processing. Trauma can feel massive and tangled, but titration helps untangle it thread by thread, letting your body digest the experience in pieces instead of all at once.

Together, pendulation and titration create a foundation for healing that's both gentle and effective. They offer a way to stay present with yourself, even in difficult moments, without feeling stuck or overwhelmed. Now, let's bring these ideas to life with an exercise designed to put them into practice.

Exercise 33: Pendulation and Titration

Now it's time to bring pendulation and titration together in a steady, intentional flow. This exercise combines the rhythmic ebb and flow of pendulation with the slow, deliberate pace of titration.

The goal here isn't to rush or force anything but to practice the art of noticing, pausing, and letting your body release tension or energy at its own pace. By taking small, manageable steps, you allow your body to adjust gradually, significantly reducing the risk of re-traumatization. This method encourages steady progress, supporting your body in releasing stored trauma while reinforcing the confidence that you can handle and process distress safely.

Try it for yourself:

1. Find a quiet, comfortable space where you won't be interrupted. Sit or lie down—whatever feels right—and let your hands rest naturally. If it feels safe, close your eyes; if not, keep them softly open, focusing on something neutral.
2. Next, think of a challenge—an emotion, a minor stressor, or a past experience that isn't too overwhelming. Allow the thought to come into focus gently.
3. Now, shift your attention to your body. Notice any sensations that arise when you think about this challenge. Do you feel tension, warmth, or heaviness? Simply observe these sensations without trying to change them. You might think, *I feel some tightness here* or *this spot feels warm*. Allow yourself to simply notice.
4. Then, turn your focus to a grounding resource—a steady sensation you're familiar with, like the weight of your feet on the floor, the feeling of your hands resting on your lap, or any other options you've identified in the last

chapter. Spend a moment here, letting this calming presence support you.
5. Begin moving your focus back and forth: Spend a few seconds noticing the challenging sensation, then return to your grounding resource for three to five deep breaths. Repeat this cycle at a pace that feels natural. If it helps, add a gentle movement or sound—a soft hum, a slight sway, or a light shake of your hands. You can use it while sitting with the distressing sensation or as you shift back to calm, helping your body process and settle into the transition.
6. When you feel stable and resourced, narrow your attention to a smaller detail of the challenging sensation—a particular place, sound, or subtle feeling connected to it. Spend a few seconds here before returning to your resource. Let your body guide the pace, keeping the shifts brief and gentle.
7. Finally, when you're ready, end the exercise by resting in your grounding resource. Take a few deep breaths and notice how your body feels now compared to when you started.

If you'd like to prepare before trying the exercise, take a moment to jot down your thoughts. This will help create a sense of direction that feels supportive. Consider these prompts:

- The challenge I want to explore is:

_____
_____
_____

- Where I notice this challenge in my body is:

- My chosen resource for grounding is:

- A small, manageable piece of the challenge I'd like to explore with titration:

After the Practice

Take a moment to reflect on your experience:

- Did the intensity of the challenge shift? If so, how?

- What did you notice about your body or emotions during the exercise?

- What insights or feelings would you like to carry forward from this practice?

_____
_____
_____

This exercise is about building trust with your body, step by step. By pairing pendulation with titration, you're giving yourself a framework to safely explore sensations without feeling stuck or overwhelmed. The more you practice, the more natural this rhythm will feel, helping you navigate challenging experiences with greater confidence and ease.

These techniques are tools you can use as you move through your day. When a stressful memory pops up out of nowhere, pendulation helps you stay with it without getting overwhelmed. If an experience feels like too much, titration lets you break it down into smaller, more manageable sensations, making it easier to process. Over time, these practices become second nature, giving you a way to move through emotions instead of feeling stuck in them.

Once these quiet moments start feeling familiar, you might find yourself wanting to take them a step further—into something more active, more fluid. That's where movement comes in. The next chapter explores how stretching, shaking, and moving your body can help you reconnect with yourself in a whole new way. Sometimes, the most powerful release doesn't come from stillness—it comes from motion. Ready to shake things up? Let's go!

9

MOVEMENT AS MEDICINE: YOGA, STRETCH AND SHAKE

Have you ever noticed how kids instinctively shake off a fall or bounce back after something scary? They'll cry, shudder, wiggle, or run to the nearest adult, but once it's out of their system, they're back to playing like nothing happened. It's almost enviable, right? Well, it's not just resilience—it's biology. Their bodies know how to reset after something overwhelming, and as adults, we still have that ability too. We've just learned to ignore it.

Instead of releasing tension, we hold onto it. Think about the ways stress sneaks into your body. Maybe it's that restless tapping of your fingers when you're overwhelmed or the way a headache starts taking shape out of nowhere. These are your body's signals, small signs that maybe something needs to move but hasn't yet had the chance.

Movement takes center stage here—not as a grueling workout or something to push through, but as a chance for your body to complete what it started. And it can be as simple as you need it to be.

Look at animals in the wild. After escaping a predator, they don't sit around rehashing the event—they shake, tremble, and move until the adrenaline clears their system. That movement is their reset button, and guess what? We have one, too. Movement engages the sensory and motor systems, helping your body process stress and recalibrate. In fact, it does more than just clear the adrenaline—physical activity also improves the functioning of the hypothalamic-pituitary-adrenal axis (HPA), that handy stress regulator of yours. It can help with sleep, boost your mood, and even aid in managing psychiatric disorders like depression and anxiety (Mahindru et al., 2023).

And if you're dealing with an injury or health condition, don't worry—movement is adaptable. It's not about perfect form; it's about finding what feels right for you. Whether you're lying down, sitting, or experimenting with gentle motions, the key is to tune into your body and follow its cues.

Ahead, we'll dive into therapeutic movements that fit seamlessly into everyday life. From subtle stretches to spontaneous shaking, these practices are designed to help your body let go and reclaim its natural rhythm. Let's begin with somatic stretching.

Simple Somatic Movements to Try at Home: Somatic Stretching

Where does your body feel tense? Where does it feel stiff? Somatic stretching is like scanning a room to figure out where the light's not quite reaching. These stretches give you a chance to pay attention to subtle shifts in tension and comfort, letting your body guide you without the pressure to get it "right."

Let's explore a few simple stretches that can help you reconnect with your body and find that sense of ease.

Exercise 34: Neck Side Stretch (Sukhasana)

Sometimes, tension builds up in your neck muscles after a long day or hours spent hunched over a desk. This stretch is a simple way to invite your body to let go. It's gentle, restorative, and easy to do anytime you need to reset.

1. Sit comfortably in a chair or on the floor and take a few deep breaths, allowing your shoulders to relax.
2. Slowly tuck your chin toward your chest, feeling the gentle stretch along the back of your neck.
3. Pause here for a moment, breathing deeply into the stretch.
4. Next, tilt your head to one side, bringing your ear toward your shoulder. Avoid forcing the movement; let it feel natural.
5. If it feels good, bring your hand from the same side your head is tilting and place it lightly on the opposite side of your head. Apply gentle pressure, just enough to deepen the stretch without discomfort.
6. To switch sides, let your head roll forward in a downward arc toward the center before tilting it to the other side.
7. Repeat this entire sequence 3–5 times, moving slowly.

In the sketch below, mark what you noticed during the stretch:

- Circle any areas where you felt tightness or tension.
- Place an X where the stretch brought the most noticeable release.
- Add words like "soft" or "cooling"—anything that can help you describe how your neck or shoulders felt during or after the stretch.

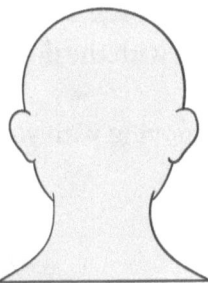

Take as much time as you need here. I encourage you to use the sketch as a tool to create a visual representation of what you're feeling physically in this moment.

Exercise 35: Bridge Pose (Setu Bandha Sarvangasana)

Some days, your back, hips, and legs feel like they're holding onto more tension than they need to—like they're gripping when they could be softening. Bridge Pose is a simple yet powerful way to counteract that tightness. It gently opens the chest, stretches the spine, and strengthens your legs, making it a great all-around reset.

1. Lie on your back with your knees bent and your feet flat on the floor, hip-width apart. Keep your arms relaxed by your sides, palms facing down.
2. Press your feet into the ground and engage your legs as you slowly lift your hips toward the ceiling. Keep your knees in line with your ankles and avoid letting them splay outward.
3. Roll your shoulders slightly underneath you to create more space in your chest. If it feels good, clasp your hands under your back for extra support.
4. Breathe deeply, holding the position for 3–5 breaths. With each inhale, feel your chest expand; with each exhale, imagine releasing tension from your lower back.

5. Slowly lower your hips back down to the ground, feeling your spine reconnect with the floor one vertebra at a time.
6. Repeat 3–5 times, moving with your breath.

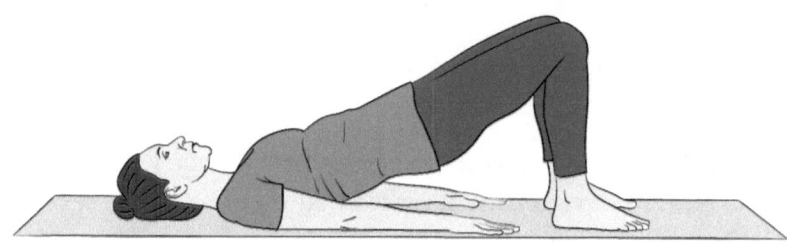

Instead of jumping up right away, take a moment to check in with your body. Gently rock your knees from side to side or hug them into your chest. What feels good right now? Where does your body naturally want to move? Let your body lead the way.

Once you're finished, take a moment to reflect on your experience:

- Did any emotions or sensations surface while holding the pose? How did the movement affect your overall state—did it bring relief, discomfort, or something unexpected?

_____
_____
_____

- After coming out of the pose, what did your body naturally want to do next? Did you follow that urge?

_____
_____
_____

Exercise 36: Supine Spinal Twist (Supta Matsyendrasana)

Think of this stretch as a reset button for your spine. It's grounding, gentle, and perfect for easing tension in your lower back.

1. Start by lying on your back with your knees bent and your feet flat on the floor. Think of this as your reset position, where you can just breathe and let your body settle.
2. Stretch your arms out to the sides, palms facing down, like you're creating a human T-shape.
3. Take a deep breath in, and as you exhale, let your knees drop to one side. Let the twist happen naturally, without forcing it. Feel what's happening in your spine and torso.
4. Hold the twist for a few breaths, noticing any shifts.
5. If you want to deepen the stretch, gently use your hand to add a little pressure to the knee, encouraging a deeper twist.
6. Slowly bring your knees back to the center as you inhale. On your next exhale, let them drop to the other side.
7. Repeat the movement 3–5 times, keeping it slow and letting your body guide you. Adjust as needed—this stretch should feel supportive, never strained.

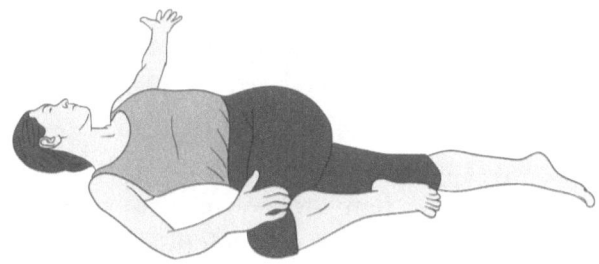

After you've completed the twist, pause and notice what your body shared with you:

- Did you notice a sensation that reminded you of a specific feeling or moment—like waking up, resting, or letting go of stress?

_____
_____
_____

- After the stretch, thank your body for what it allowed you to feel. Write down one thing you appreciate about your spine, back, or overall movement.

_____
_____
_____

Exercise 37: Reclined Pigeon Pose (Supta Kapotasana)

Your hips do a lot for you. They carry you through long days of sitting, standing, or walking, they take on more than they let on. When tension builds, it can feel like stiffness, restriction, or even an achy tightness that lingers. Reclined Pigeon Pose is a gentle way to unlock some of that built-up tension and bring mobility back to your hips.

1. Lie on your back with your knees bent and feet flat on the floor. Keep your spine relaxed and your breath steady.
2. Lift your right foot and place your right ankle over your left thigh, just above the knee. Let your right knee fall outward, forming a figure-four shape with your legs.
3. Thread your hands behind your left thigh, interlacing your fingers. If this feels too intense, keep your left foot on the ground. If you'd like a deeper stretch, gently pull your left thigh toward your chest.

4. Breathe deeply as you hold the position, letting your right hip release with each exhale. Stay here for 20–30 seconds, noticing where you feel the stretch.
5. Slowly release your left thigh and lower your right foot back to the ground. Repeat on the other side, placing your left ankle over your right thigh and following the same steps.

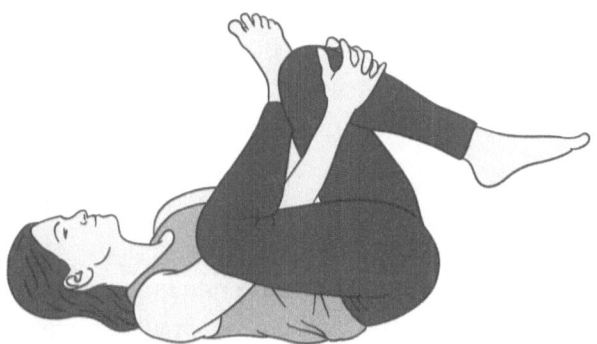

Once you've completed this stretch, take a moment to reflect:

- **Circle** the side where you felt the most tension—was it your right hip, left hip, or lower back?
- Imagine your hips are gears in a machine. How smoothly did they feel like they were turning before and after the exercise? Reflect on the change.

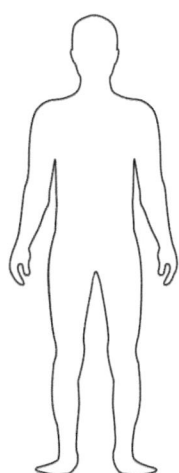

_____

_____

_____

Stretching is a great first step toward releasing the tension your body holds, but it's only the beginning. As you stretch, you might feel your body craving more fluid movements or a deeper connection between breath and motion. Yoga offers the perfect next step, blending strength and flow to deepen your connection to your body and release what no longer serves you. Let's take a look.

Simple Somatic Movements to Try at Home: Somatic Yoga

Think of yoga as the art of moving and breathing with intention. Each movement, paired with intentional breathing, taps into your parasympathetic nervous system and helps you flip the switch from "go-go-go" mode to "it's safe to breathe again."

I learned this during one of the most frustrating chapters of my life: my battle with relentless migraines. At one point, it felt like I was living in a loop—barely recovering from one migraine before the next would slam into me. My world became smaller, revolving around trying to manage the pain. Desperate for something, *anything*, to help, I turned to yoga. Not for the migraines specifically, but because I needed a way to calm my mind and feel like I had some control over my day.

I started small—just 10 minutes every morning. No elaborate poses, no expectations. To my surprise, by the end of that month, I'd only had one migraine. I was shocked. I hadn't changed anything else in my routine, yet this simple practice seemed to have an effect I couldn't ignore. That experience taught me that yoga didn't just calm my mind, it helped my body process and release the tension it had been holding onto for who knows how long.

This is the essence of yoga in somatic therapy. It's not about perfecting a pose or muscling through discomfort—it's about listening. Your body has a story to tell, and every stretch, twist, and breath is a chance to hear it. Maybe in a Seated Forward Bend, you feel a gentle stretch unraveling along your spine. Or in Child's Pose, your shoulders finally drop, and your breath slows like an exhalation you didn't know you were holding. Even research is starting to catch up

—studies show that yoga can help release trauma stored in the body, being particularly helpful for those who carry the weight of early traumatic experiences (Vancampfort et al., 2012).

Ready to explore it for yourself? Let's dive into a simple yoga sequence you can do right at home. No fancy props, no experience needed—just a bit of space and a willingness to listen to your body.

Exercise 38: Child's Pose (Balasana)

This pose is like a full-body sigh—a chance to let everything settle and reconnect with your breath.

1. Start by kneeling on the floor, sitting back on your heels.
2. Fold forward, letting your forehead rest gently on the mat or a cushion.
3. Stretch your arms out in front of you, or let them rest alongside your body with your palms facing up.
4. Breathe deeply, feeling your back expand with each inhale and soften with each exhale.
5. Stay here for as long as it feels good, letting your body sink into the support of the ground.

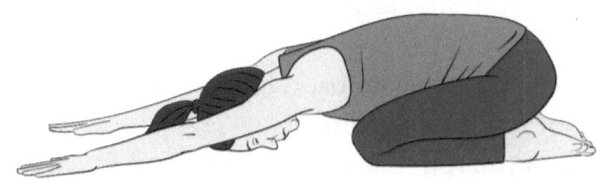

As you rest here, let your attention drift inward. These quiet moments are opportunities to notice what's happening beneath the surface. Here's a fun way to explore what your body is telling you:

- Take a moment to notice how each part of your body feels. Write one word that describes how each of them

feels—whether it's tight, soft, heavy, light, or anything else that comes to mind:
- **Back:** _____
- **Neck:** _____
- **Shoulders:** _____
- **Arms:** _____
- **Legs:** _____
- **Breath:** _____

• Now that you've described each area, take a moment to reflect. What do these words say about your overall state right now?

_____

_____

_____

Exercise 39: Cat-Cow Pose (Marjaryasana to Bitilasana)

This gentle movement helps release tension in your spine and creates a rhythm between your breath and your body.

1. Come onto your hands and knees, with your wrists in line with your shoulders and your knees in line with your hips.
2. Inhale as you arch your back, lifting your head and tailbone toward the ceiling (Cow Pose).
3. Exhale as you round your spine, tucking your chin toward your chest and drawing your belly in (Cat Pose).
4. Move slowly between these two poses, matching your breath to your movement.
5. Repeat for 5–10 breaths, noticing how your spine feels as you flow.

MOVEMENT AS MEDICINE: YOGA, STRETCH AND SHAKE

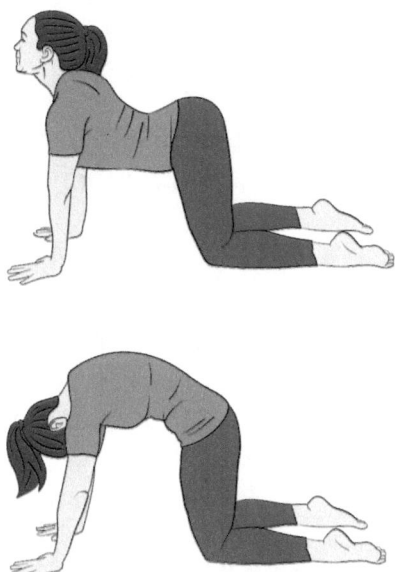

The flow between the Cat and Cow Pose gives you a moment to notice where tension lingers and where release begins. As you finish the stretch, sit back for a moment and reflect:

- Does your spine feel looser or more mobile than when you started? Where do you still notice tension, if any?

_____
_____
_____

- If you had to describe the sensation in your spine right now, what words come to mind? You can use a metaphor, an image, or just describe the physical feeling.

_____
_____
_____

Exercise 40: Seated Forward Bend Pose (Pashchimottanasana)

This pose invites you to release tension in your back and legs, offering a moment to tune into the sensations in your body.

1. Sit on the floor with your legs extended straight in front of you.
2. Inhale as you lengthen your spine, reaching your arms overhead.
3. Exhale as you fold forward, letting your hands rest on your legs, feet, or the floor.
4. Let gravity guide you, keeping your movements soft and your breath steady.
5. Hold the pose for 5–10 breaths, noticing what feels tight or where you can soften.

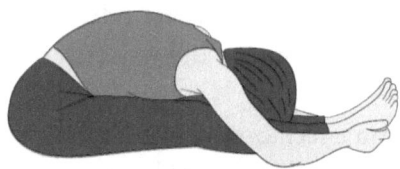

There's no need to force anything—let gravity guide you and notice how your body naturally responds. After the stretch, sit upright and take a moment to reflect on:

- What part of your body feels the most different after the stretch—your back, legs, or hips? Write down any sensations or observations.

_____
_____
_____

Exercise 41: Corpse Pose (Savasana)

This is your moment to completely let go and let your body absorb the benefits of your practice. It's not about doing anything—just being.

1. Lie on your back with your arms resting at your sides, palms facing up.
2. Let your legs relax and fall open naturally.
3. Close your eyes and take slow, deep breaths, noticing the weight of your body sinking into the mat.
4. Stay here for as long as you'd like, allowing your breath to flow naturally.

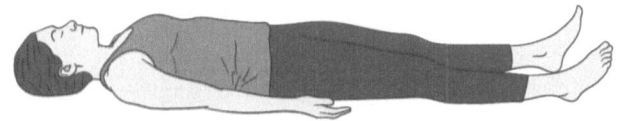

In this stillness, let yourself be curious about what your body is telling you. This is a time to listen, as your body settles into rest. If you'd like, imagine a color that represents how your body feels in this moment and answer:

- What color comes to mind?
  _____
- Why do you think this color represents your current state?

_____
_____
_____

Yoga teaches you to find harmony between stillness and movement, offering a chance to reconnect with your body through mindful awareness.

But there are times when your body doesn't just want calm—it craves release. Next, we'll explore the power of uninhibited movement as a way to let go of tension and rediscover the freedom within you.

Dance, Shake, and Release: Moving Through Emotion

If somatic yoga feels like a calm, flowing stream, dance and shaking are like a wild jam session—unpredictable, freeing, and full of life. And here's the cool part: It's not just fun, it's effective. Studies show that dancing can significantly reduce PTSD symptoms (Koch et al., 2014) and help trauma survivors reconnect with their bodies, improving both body image and a sense of comfort in their skin (Karkou & Meekums, 2017).

So, why does it work? When you move freely—whether it's a full-on dance party in your living room or a few minutes of shaking—you're giving your body a chance to release not just stress, but any built-up tension, anxiety, frustration, or even grief that might be lingering. It's not about being perfect or following some unwritten dance rules. It's about letting go—physically, emotionally, and maybe even mentally.

And the best part? There's no right or wrong way to do it. No one's watching, no one's judging your moves. It's just you, your body, and the rhythm (whether it's music or silence—whatever feels right). Let's dive into some simple exercises to help you shake off what's been weighing you down and feel more at ease.

Exercise 42: Shake It Off

Shaking is one of the simplest ways to let go of tension and reset your nervous system. Whether you're feeling overwhelmed or just stuck in a funk, this playful practice helps you shake off what's weighing you down—literally.

1. Stand in a spot where you can move freely without worrying about bumping into anything. Feel your feet grounded on the floor.
2. Start small. Gently shake one part of your body—your hands, one arm, or maybe a leg. Keep the movement loose and light.
3. Gradually involve your whole body. Let the shakes spread naturally to your arms, torso, and head. If it feels good, let the movement grow bigger and bouncier, adding more energy.
4. Go wild if you're up for it! Let your entire body move freely, swaying or bouncing lightly on your feet. You can even add sound—hum, sigh, or laugh if it feels right.
5. After 2–3 minutes, slow the movement down. Stand still and take a few deep breaths.

Now that you've slowed down, take a moment to tune into how your body feels. Shaking creates a natural rhythm, and capturing this experience can help you connect with the shifts in your body.

- Complete the following sentences to describe your experience:
    - The part of my body that felt the most alive during shaking was _____.
    - Shaking felt like _____. (e.g., letting go of a weight, buzzing energy, waking up).
    - My body surprised me when _____.
    - Right now, I feel _____ compared to when I started.

Exercise 43: Dance It Out

Dancing is about feeling good. Whether you're processing emotions or just boosting your mood, this practice helps you reconnect with your body in a way that's both fun and freeing. If you've ever watched *Grey's Anatomy*, you might remember Meredith and Cristina's "dance it out" moments—shaking off stress, grief, or just a long day with music and movement. Let that be your inspiration as you explore how dancing can be a tool for healing.

1. Start by choosing your music. Pick something that matches your mood—a song with a beat that lifts you up, or something slower and soulful.
   - No music? No problem. Dance to the rhythm of your breath or the sounds around you.
   - If you'd like a visual aid to start, you can try a somatic dancing video or a class.
2. Stand still for a moment, feeling your feet on the ground. Let the music (or silence) wash over you. Breathe deeply, giving your body time to tune in.
3. Begin moving in a way that feels natural. Maybe it's swaying side to side, tapping your feet, or rolling your shoulders. Let the rhythm and your body guide you.
4. Expand your movement gradually. Let your entire body join the dance, whether that means big sweeping motions or subtle shifts. There's no wrong way—just follow what feels good.
5. When the song ends, pause. Stand still or sit down and notice any changes in your body or emotions.

Take a moment to pause after the music stops. Let your body settle and notice how you're feeling. This is a time to reflect on the freedom and energy you just experienced.

In a few sentences, write about your dance. Imagine describing it to a friend:

- What did the movement feel like? Was it smooth, wild, or something else?

_____

_____

_____

- Did any emotions bubble up while you danced? Joy, release, or even something unexpected?

_____

_____

_____

After dancing and shaking, your body has had the chance to release tension and rediscover its freedom. But sometimes your body might crave something gentler, a practice that brings calm and focus while still inviting you to move with intention.

Qigong: Cultivating Vitality Through Movement

Qigong is like meditation's more active, free-spirited cousin—the one that doesn't just sit still but moves, breathes, and tunes into energy in a way that feels both grounding and refreshing. This ancient Chinese practice has been around for thousands of years, blending smooth movements, focused breathing, and meditation to create a powerful balance of energy and peace (Choi, 2024).

Now, let's put this knowledge into action. Here are two simple Qigong exercises you can try right now.

Exercise 44: The Gathering Breath

This practice is a gentle way to center yourself and replenish your energy, especially during moments of stress or fatigue. Think of it as gathering the good stuff from the world around you and bringing it into your body.

1. Stand tall with your feet hip-width apart, knees slightly bent, and arms relaxed at your sides. Let your shoulders soften and imagine your body rooted to the ground like a strong, steady tree.
2. As you inhale deeply through your nose, slowly raise your arms in a wide, graceful arc above your head. Picture yourself gathering positive energy from the space around you—like scooping light or warmth from the air.
3. Exhale gently through your mouth, lowering your arms back down with your palms facing your body. Imagine the energy you've gathered flowing down through you, grounding you into the earth.
4. Repeat this movement 5–10 times, letting your breath and arms move together in harmony.

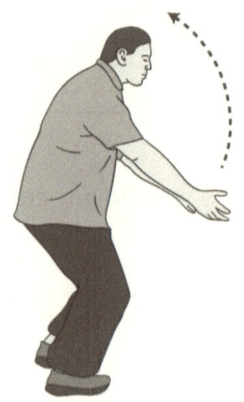

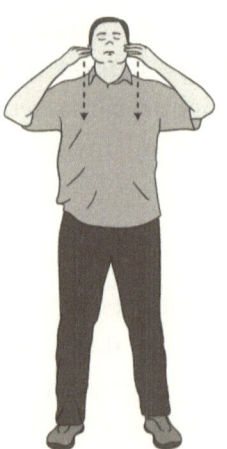

As you finish, let the energy settle and take a moment to reflect using the prompts below to describe your experience. Think of it as jotting down a quick snapshot of how this practice felt:

- As I raised my arms, I imagined gathering _____.

- The energy settled in my
  _____.
- This practice made me feel more
  _____.
- If I could describe this moment in one word, it would be
  _____.

Exercise 45: Swaying Tree

This practice is all about finding balance and releasing tension. Imagine yourself as a tree, firmly rooted but free to move with the breeze—steady, fluid, and connected.

1. Stand with your feet slightly wider than hip-width apart and your knees soft. Distribute your weight evenly, feeling your feet press firmly into the ground. Visualize your feet as roots growing deep into the earth, holding you steady.
2. Begin to gently sway by shifting your weight from one foot to the other. Keep the movement slow and fluid, as if you're moving with a soft, rhythmic breeze.
3. Sync your breath with your movement. Inhale as you shift to one side, exhale as you flow to the other. Let the rhythm of your breath guide the sway.
4. Gradually let the swaying become smaller and slower until you return to stillness. Pause here, noticing how your body feels—grounded, calm, or energized.

As you come to stillness, take a moment to soak in the experience. Let your body and mind settle, and imagine you're writing a note to your future self—a little reminder of how it felt to sway, breathe, and let go:

> *Dear Future Me,*
> *After the Swaying Tree practice, my body felt*
> *_____, and my breath became*
> *_____. This moment reminded*
> *me that_____.*

Keep this note as a reminder of your strength and balance.

These small moments add up, shaping the way you move through your day—literally and figuratively. It's less about squeezing in a workout and more about creating a rhythm that keeps you feeling present, at ease, and in sync with yourself. The more you listen to your body's cues, the more natural these movements become, like a conversation unfolding without words.

But movement is just one way to reconnect. Touch adds another dimension, offering a sense of safety, grounding, and self-support. When used intentionally, it becomes a tool for soothing, healing, and deepening the dialogue between body and mind. In the next chapter, we'll explore somatic touch and self-soothing techniques designed to help you feel more connected and whole.

10

HEAL THROUGH SOMATIC TOUCH: SELF-SOOTHING TECHNIQUES

IMAGINE you're sitting with a close friend, anxiously waiting for an important phone call—maybe news about a job offer, test results, or something that could change everything. Your chest feels tight, and your thoughts are running in circles. Then, your friend reaches over and gives your hand a gentle squeeze. No words, no big gestures—just that small, steady pressure. And somehow, it helps. You exhale, your shoulders drop just a little, and for a moment, you feel less alone in the waiting. That's the quiet magic of touch. From day one, it's been our built-in survival tool, a way to feel secure, grounded, and connected.

Why? Because safe touch triggers the release of oxytocin—the hormone that builds trust, connection, and relaxation (The Science of Hugs, 2023). It's also a natural stress reliever, lowering cortisol levels and activating your parasympathetic nervous system, the part that signals, "You're safe. You can breathe." As your brain gets the message, your heart rate slows, the tension eases, and that sense of fight, flight, or freeze starts to fade, making room for calm to take its place.

If you're carrying trauma, though, touch might feel less like a comfort and more like an unknown territory. Instead of plunging in headfirst, it's about easing in, finding what feels doable. Maybe that's pressing your palms together, or simply noticing the weight of your hands resting in your lap. Safe touch becomes a bridge, helping you reconnect with your body in a way that feels right for you.

Now that we recognize *how* touch influences both body and mind, the next question is: What exactly does it do for you? Let's explore how somatic touch can help you improve your physical, mental, and emotional well-being.

Benefits of Somatic Touch

Safe touch does more than just help you relax—though let's be honest, that's a pretty great perk. It isn't just about feeling good—it has a way of working on a deeper level, bringing a whole range of benefits along with it:

- **Brings you back to the present:** Ever felt like you're physically here, but mentally off in another universe—like you're trying to sort out your finances or making a list of everything you need to get ready for the kids for school tomorrow? Safe touch helps pull you back, grounding you in the moment.
- **Heals early attachment wounds:** Touch is one of the first ways we learn connection, which is why it plays a key role in healing attachment-related trauma (Davis et al., 2017). Safe, nonjudgmental contact can help rebuild trust—not just in others, but in yourself.
- **Boosts your awareness:** Safe touch sharpens interception, your ability to tune into what's happening inside your body. Maybe you start picking up on the subtle shift in your posture when you're feeling uneasy, or how your stomach tightens slightly when you agree to something you don't actually want to do. The more you tune in, the easier it becomes to understand these signals and take action—whether it's adjusting your stance,

HEAL THROUGH SOMATIC TOUCH: SELF-SOOTHING TECHN... 135

taking a deep breath, or setting a boundary before discomfort turns into stress.

Armed with this knowledge, the next step is figuring out how to bring more of it into your life. Let's explore some ways you can tap into the benefits of somatic touch—starting now.

Somatic Touch in Action: Self-Holding and Self-Soothing Techniques

These simple exercises are designed to help you reconnect with your body and bring a little calm into your day. No special tools, no complicated steps—just your hands and a few quiet moments of self-care.

Exercise 46: The Two-Step Self-Holding Exercise

Imagine you're lying in bed, scrolling through your phone, telling yourself you'll put it down in just one more minute. Except that minute turns into 10, and instead of winding down, your mind is buzzing with everything you didn't get done today. This simple practice helps quiet the mental static and brings you back to the present. Whether you're feeling restless, overwhelmed, or just disconnected from yourself, it's a quick way to reset and find a sense of calm.

Let's look into it:

1. Sit or lie down in a way that feels good. If closing your eyes helps you focus, go for it. Otherwise, keep a soft gaze.
2. Place one hand on your forehead and the other on your heart. Let them rest naturally. If you're lying

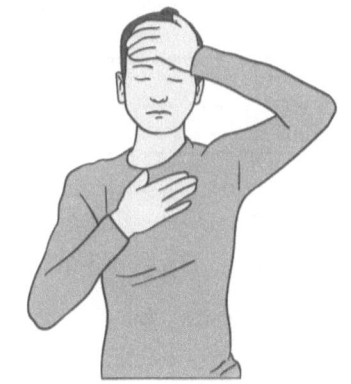

down, support your arm with a pillow so you can stay relaxed.

3. Focus on the space between your hands. Simply notice what you feel between them—warmth, coolness, energy, or even nothing at all. Stay here for a few moments, allowing your body to settle.

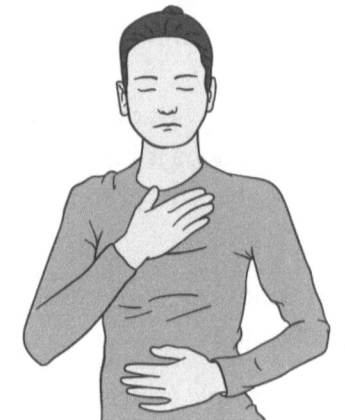

4. When you're ready, move your top hand to your belly. Rest it there and bring your attention to the space between your hands again. Does anything shift? Maybe your breath slows down, or your body softens a little.
5. Gently release the hold. Lift your hands and place them on your lap or by your sides. Take a deep breath and notice how you feel now. Open your eyes if they were closed, stretch if you want to, and give yourself a moment before moving on with your day.

Afterward, imagine your body could send you a note in response. Complete this sentence:

- I thank myself for this moment. It helped me feel

_____

_____

_____

Exercise 47: The Gentle Hand Technique

Now imagine you're standing in the checkout line, shifting your weight from one foot to the other while your mind runs through a mental checklist—did you grab everything? Will you make it home in time to cook? Did that text you sent earlier come across the wrong way? Your body feels tense, but you're not sure why. This is when a simple touch—warm, steady, and intentional—can help redirect that restless energy, giving your nervous system the signal it needs to settle.

Here's how to try it:

1. Rub your hands together until they feel warm. Pay attention to the tingling or heat that builds as you move.
2. Place your warm hands on your face, neck, or shoulders —wherever they're needed most. Let the warmth settle into your muscles and notice how your body responds.

Afterward, take a moment to reflect:

- What area did your hands gravitate to the most? Why do you think that was?

_____
_____
_____

- How did your body respond to the warmth and pressure? Did the tension ease, or did you notice any resistance?

_____
_____
_____

Exercise 48: The Rock-and-Breathe Hug

Some days, it feels like the world is coming at you all at once— everything's fast, loud, and just a bit too much. Maybe you wish you had someone nearby to give you a comforting hug. But you can give yourself that same feeling of comfort, even when you're alone.

This exercise uses the natural rhythm of gentle rocking to tap into your body's self-soothing abilities, helping you feel grounded and held.

Let's explore it step by step:

1. Find a comfortable spot—sit on a chair or the floor, or even stand if that feels right.
2. Cross your arms over your chest, resting your hands on opposite shoulders. Notice the weight of your arms as they settle around you.

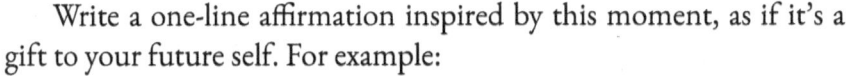

3. Begin to gently rock from side to side, pairing the movement with slow, deep breaths. Let the rhythm bring a sense of ease.
4. As you move, imagine you're holding yourself the way you would a close friend. What would you want them to feel in this moment? Offer yourself the same.

Write a one-line affirmation inspired by this moment, as if it's a gift to your future self. For example:

- "I am always here for myself."
- "This moment is mine to breathe and be."
- Your turn:

_____
_____
_____

These exercises show us that sometimes the most comforting touch can come from our own hands. But self-soothing isn't the only way to experience the benefits of touch—sometimes, a little extra support can make all the difference. When intentional pressure is applied in just the right way, it can signal safety to the nervous system.

The Weighted Blanket Effect

The weighted blanket is a perfect example of this principle—a cozy, full-body hug you didn't know you needed. Based on deep pressure stimulation (the same reason swaddling calms babies or a firm hug feels so grounding), these blankets help settle the nervous system and create a deep sense of security.

And they do more than just feel cozy. The gentle, even pressure encourages the release of serotonin, your mood booster, and melatonin, your natural sleep aid, while lowering the stress hormone that keeps you wired when you'd rather be winding down (Noyed, 2023).

A meta-analysis found that weighted blankets can also reduce anxiety, especially for people managing conditions like depression, bipolar disorder, ADHD, and autism. In fact, participants who used weighted blankets saw a 47% reduction in anxiety symptoms compared to those who didn't (Wong et al., 2024). That's a big shift for something as simple as an extra layer of pressure.

Whether you use one to decompress after a long day or to create a sense of security during moments of stress, the right amount of pressure can be a game-changer. It's not a magic fix, but for many, it makes relaxation feel more accessible and comfort more immediate.

While self-touch and self-soothing are powerful, there's something special about the warmth of a trusted hand. Shared touch can strengthen connection, build a sense of safety, and offer comfort in a way that feels different to the solo techniques we explored. Let's dive into some partnered exercises that bring grounding, care, and a little extra support.

Partner Exercises for Safe and Supportive Touch

When we hear the word "partner," it's easy to think of a romantic relationship. But in this case, a partner can be anyone you trust—a close friend, a family member, or someone who makes you feel safe and supported. Touch, when shared with care and mutual consent, has a way of strengthening bonds and creating a sense of calm.

Let's start with something simple.

Exercise 49: The Hand Dance

If you've ever watched *The Vampire Diaries*, you might remember the famous Founder's Day Ball dance between Elena and Damon—a wordless, magnetic connection that speaks volumes. Now, picture yourself sitting in a quiet room with your partner or someone you trust, but something feels a little off. Maybe your mind is still holding on to a stressful conversation or the busy moments of the day. You want to connect with them, but words don't feel quite right. The Hand Dance is an easy way to do this—it helps you tune in to each other's energy without needing to talk, allowing you both to feel the presence of the other in a simple, subtle way.

1. Sit across from your partner in a comfortable spot. Raise your hands and hold them just an inch apart, palm to palm.
2. Without touching, begin to move your hands slowly. Let one of you take the lead, and the other follows, like a quiet, improvised dance.
3. Notice the subtle sensations between your hands—heat, tingling, or even a gentle pull. Switch roles after a minute, letting the other person guide.

Once you've finished, take a moment to reflect together:

- How effective did this exercise feel in helping you connect and feel supported without physical touch?

_____
_____
_____

- Describe the sensations you felt between your hands—did you notice warmth, tingling, or something else?

_____
_____
_____

- Complete this sentence together:
  - Moving without touching felt _____ because _____.

Exercise 50: Dynamic Cuddles

Now imagine you're at home, feeling emotionally drained from the day. You want comfort but don't feel like settling into a quiet, still embrace. Maybe you're restless, or perhaps you just need a bit of space to adjust while still feeling held. Dynamic Cuddles can be the perfect practice for this—providing the warmth of touch while giving you the freedom to move and shift in a way that feels right for your body in the moment.

1. Sit or lie down together in a position that feels comfortable for both of you. This could be sitting back-to-back, lying side by side, or one person resting their head on the other's lap.
2. Begin to explore gentle movements, like swaying side to

side or rocking slightly forward and back. Let the motion feel intuitive and relaxed.
3. Communicate as you go. Ask, "Does this feel okay?" or "Would you like me to adjust?" The goal is to find a shared rhythm that feels good for both of you.

Afterward, take a few moments to check in with each other:

- Is there a part of your body that feels lighter or more relaxed now than before?

_____
_____
_____

- Did you notice any areas of tension or resistance while we moved? How did that feel?

_____
_____
_____

When shared with trust, touch becomes its own kind of conversation. A steady hand, a reassuring squeeze, the quiet presence of someone nearby—all of it communicates safety and connection. But sometimes, the comfort your body craves requires your own hands to get to work. Let's explore how self-massage can become a tool for grounding, relaxation, and healing.

The Therapeutic Power of Massage

Looking for another way to experience somatic touch? Massage is your answer. It offers a wealth of benefits, from reconnecting you with your body and releasing tension to even supporting your emotional balance. For example, a study of 68 individuals with

Generalized Anxiety Disorder (GAD) showed that therapeutic massage significantly reduced anxiety, with participants experiencing a 50% decrease in their Hamilton Anxiety Rating Scale (HARS) scores compared to control groups (Sherman et al., 2010).

The best part? You don't need an hour-long session at a spa to feel the benefits. With just a few simple techniques, you can tap into the power of massage on your own. Here are two easy ways to start.

Exercise 51: Neck and Shoulder Tension Release

Stress loves to hang out in your neck and shoulders. This quick self-massage can help you send it packing.

1. Sit in a comfortable chair or on the edge of your bed. Let your back rest naturally and take a few deep breaths, imagining your shoulders dropping away from your ears as you exhale.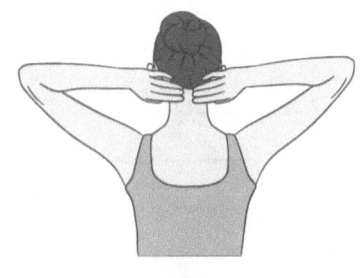
2. Place your fingertips on the back of your neck, just below the base of your skull. Begin to make small, circular motions, applying gentle pressure as you move down 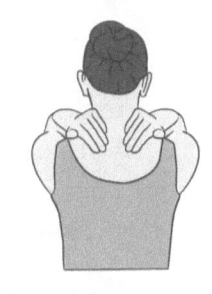 the sides of your neck. Pause and breathe into any spots that feel extra tight.
3. Shift your focus to your shoulders. Place your hands on top and use your thumbs to knead into the muscles. Roll your thumbs outward along the curve of your shoulders, paying special attention to any areas that feel tense.
4. Let your breath guide you—inhale as you apply gentle pressure, exhale as you release. Notice how the rhythm of your breath supports your movements.

5. Continue for 5–10 minutes, adjusting pressure and pace as needed.

As you finish, take a moment to notice the difference:

- Where did you feel the most tension before starting? How does it feel now?

_____
_____
_____

- Did your breathing change as you worked through the massage?

_____
_____
_____

Exercise 52: Full-Body Relaxation With a Tool

If you want to take self-massage up a notch, adding a tool—like a foam roller or massage ball—can help target tension more precisely. Whether it's your back, legs, or feet, this technique helps you find those stubborn tight spots and work through them in a more focused way.

1. Pick your tool. A foam roller, massage ball, or even a rolled-up towel will do. Find a space where you can move freely, whether it's lying on the floor or sitting in a supportive chair.
2. Focus on one area at a time:
    - **For your back:** Lie down and place the foam roller under your upper back. Slowly roll up and down, pausing on tight spots.

- **For your legs:** Sit with your legs extended and the roller or ball under one thigh. Roll slowly back and forth, keeping the movement controlled, and then repeat on the other leg.
- **For your feet:** Sit or stand with a massage ball under one foot. Press down gently and roll it under your arch, heel, and toes, and then repeat on the other foot.

3. Tune into what you feel. Notice areas that feel tight, tender, or unexpectedly tense. Pause on those spots and take a few deep breaths, letting your body relax into the pressure.
4. Continue for 5–10 minutes, shifting to different areas as needed.

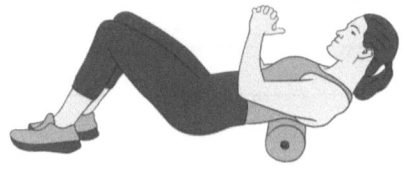

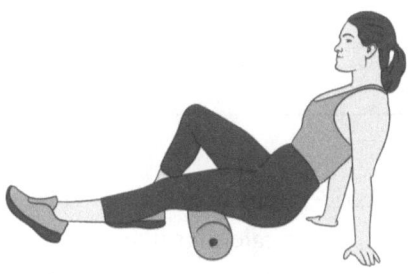

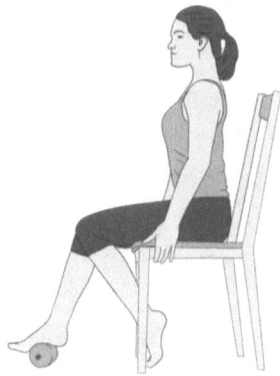

Once you're done, reflect for a moment:

- Which areas felt the tightest when you started?

_____
_____
_____

- Did you notice any shifts or releases?

_____
_____
_____

Massage and somatic touch don't have to be occasional luxuries you need to pencil into your calendar like a dentist appointment, nor should they be reserved for those rare self-care Sundays that never quite happen the way you intend. It works best when you include it in the little moments that already shape your day.

Still, some sensations don't let go so easily. It's like a song stuck in your head—one you didn't choose and can't seem to turn off. That's because your nervous system isn't just responding to *right now*; it's running on old data, shaped by every experience that came before. Touch can send signals of safety, but if your body is still tuned into past stress, those signals might not land the way you'd expect.

So, how do you change the track? That's where understanding your nervous system makes all the difference. In the next chapter, we'll explore Polyvagal Theory—how it explains those lingering sensations and why some emotions or body responses stick around long after the moment has passed. More importantly, we'll dive into how you can work with your nervous system to gently shift those patterns, making space for regulation, safety, and ease.

11

RESET AND RESTORE: POLYVAGAL THEORY AND VAGAL NERVE REGULATION

IN THIS LAST CHAPTER, we return to the vagus nerve—the body's internal messenger we met back in Chapter 2. It plays a key role in keeping everything in sync between your brain and vital organs. But this nerve is more than just background support; it's the star in your body's drama, deciding if you feel calm, on edge, or shut down.

The vagus nerve is the tenth cranial nerve, and its name—Latin for "wandering"—fits perfectly because it roams all over your body. Starting at the medulla oblongata in the brainstem, it meanders through your throat, heart, lungs, and digestive system. If your body were a city, the vagus nerve would be its main highway, linking key neighborhoods and keeping traffic flowing.

More than just a traveler, it's the regulator that decides if you feel safe and connected or stuck on high alert. Thankfully, the vagus nerve is incredibly adaptable. With the right tools, you can help it regain flexibility and settle into a calmer rhythm. Let's break down the Polyvagal Theory to understand how the vagus nerve interacts with the rest of your nervous system and how you can influence it.

Understanding the Polyvagal Theory

Your somatic toolkit is full of ways to connect with your body—grounding exercises, breathwork, resourcing—but have you ever wondered why some sensations seem to linger? Or why certain emotions feel stuck on repeat, even after you've done all the right things? Polyvagal Theory is the tool to decode your nervous system's patterns, showing how it moves between safety, stress, and shutdown—and why the shifts between states matter for healing.

Developed by Dr. Stephen Porges, a renowned neuroscientist and expert in the field of trauma and stress, Polyvagal Theory explains that your autonomic nervous system isn't just about fight, flight, or freeze (Clarke, 2019). It's constantly scanning your surroundings through a process called neuroception—an unconscious check-in that determines whether you feel safe or at risk. This scan happens beneath your awareness, shaping everything from your mood to how you respond in daily interactions.

Your nervous system works within three primary states:

- **Ventral vagal:** When your body senses safety, this system is in charge. Your breath is steady, your heart rate is balanced, and you feel engaged, present, and open to connection.
- **Sympathetic:** As we discussed in previous chapters, when your nervous system detects a challenge, it quickly shifts into fight, flight, or freeze mode. Your heart rate increases, muscles tense, and adrenaline surges through your body to help you respond. While this reaction is useful for short bursts, it can be exhausting if it becomes your default state.
- **Dorsal vagal:** When stress becomes overwhelming and your system doesn't see an escape, it pulls the emergency brake. Energy drains, breathing slows, and everything feels distant or muted.

These shifts follow a hierarchy, prioritizing connection first. But if trauma has disrupted the system, it can leave you feeling stuck, bouncing between anxiety and exhaustion or shutting down when things feel too much. Even in moments where there's no real danger, your nervous system might still be bracing for impact.

This explains why some regulation techniques work wonders one day and fall flat the next. The trick isn't just knowing what to do—it's knowing when to do it.

The Window of Tolerance

Your ability to self-regulate hinges on whether you're inside or outside your Window of Tolerance. Coined by Dr. Dan Siegel, this concept describes that sweet spot where your nervous system can handle stress without tipping into overwhelm or shutting down (Wright, 2022). When you're operating inside this window, you can think clearly, process emotions effectively, and face challenges without feeling like you're drowning.

But we know life isn't always so accommodating. When stress, trauma, or daily pressures push you outside this window, you land in one of two dysregulated states:

- **Hyperarousal:** Your system overloads. You feel wired, anxious, restless, or irritable. Thoughts race, your body refuses to settle, and everything feels like too much.
- **Hypoarousal:** In contrast, your system shuts down. You feel sluggish, emotionally distant, and disconnected—as if you're just going through the motions instead of fully experiencing life.

This is where Polyvagal Theory ties it all together. When you're stuck in hyperarousal, your body is likely on sympathetic overdrive—too much energy with no outlet. Conversely, if you're in hypoarousal, you've probably slipped into dorsal vagal shutdown, where your system conserves energy by numbing out (Porges, 2022).

When your Window of Tolerance is narrow, even small stressors can push you over the edge (Wright, 2022). This is why some days, a deep breath works like magic, and other days, it feels useless. If you're too activated, breathwork might not be enough—you might need movement, sound, or touch. If you're in shutdown, stillness can make it worse, and gentle activation (like rocking or humming) might be what helps bring you back.

Recognizing where you are in your nervous system at any given moment helps you pick the right tool instead of feeling stuck in trial-and-error mode. And that's exactly what we're going to practice now.

Rewiring Relaxation With Vagus Nerve Regulation: Techniques

We've unpacked the science, mapped out the nervous system's quirks, and explored why some days you're as cool as a cucumber and others you're one email away from a meltdown. Now, it's time to put that knowledge to work. The following exercises are practical, tangible ways to nudge your nervous system toward regulation and help relaxation feel less like a fluke and more like something you can cultivate.

Exercise 53: Tracking Your Nervous System

A great way to understand how your nervous system is doing is to track it—kind of like checking the weather before heading outside. Is it stormy with stress? Clear skies with calm? Or a bit unpredictable? This practice helps you tune into the subtle signals your body is sending so you can respond with more awareness and care.

1. Find a quiet space, sit comfortably, and take a few slow breaths. Think of it as a quick "status check" before jumping into your day.
2. Notice how you're breathing—deep and steady, or shallow and tight? Are your muscles relaxed or bracing

like you're about to dodge a flying dodgeball? Check your temperature, heart rate, and general sense of ease.
3. Check your emotional state. Are you feeling restless? Stuck? Energized? Calm? Your emotions give you clues about where your nervous system is hanging out.
4. Identify your zone:
   - Feeling wired, jumpy, or like you're ready to fight a bear? You're likely in sympathetic activation (fight or flight).
   - Feeling sluggish, foggy, or like your couch might swallow you whole? That's dorsal vagal shutdown (freeze mode).
   - Feeling engaged, present, and safe? You're in ventral vagal regulation (social engagement mode).
5. If you're stuck in stress or shutdown, try a small regulation move to activate your vagus nerve. You'll find some of these techniques below to help guide your system back to balance.

Now that you've taken this internal snapshot, let's decode what it means for you:

- What patterns in your body's signals surprised you the most?

_____
_____
_____

Exercise 54: Expanding Your Window of Tolerance

So, we know that some days, stress rolls off you like water off a raincoat. Other days, a single email or a weird look from a stranger is enough to send you spiraling. This exercise is designed to strengthen your ability to stay present and regulated, even when life gets unpredictable.

Let's get started:

1. Sit or lie down somewhere quiet and take a few deep breaths. Let your body settle.
2. Check your current state: Do you feel antsy and wired? Disconnected and foggy? Or are you somewhere in that sweet spot of feeling present and balanced? Just notice without judgment.
3. Think of something recently that was slightly stressful but not a total disaster—like dealing with a snippy email or a delayed bus.
4. Observe your body's response: Does your breath get shallow? Do your muscles tighten up? Maybe your stomach knots just a little? Stay with the sensations for a few moments without trying to change them.
5. Now, try a small regulating action—lengthen your exhale, shake out your hands, or recall a comforting memory as we explored in Chapter 7. The goal is to see if you can remain present without being overwhelmed.

After completing the exercise, reflect on your experience:

- Can you describe any changes you noticed in your ability to stay present with discomfort?

_____
_____
_____

- What specific small action helped you maintain balance within your Window of Tolerance?

_____

_____

_____

Exercise 55: Progressive Muscle Relaxation (PMR)

Stress doesn't always announce itself with flashing lights—it tends to settle quietly into your muscles, tightening its grip until you realize your shoulders are up by your ears. This exercise helps you track down that hidden tension and let it go, one breath, one muscle at a time.

1. Sit or lie down in a quiet place where you won't be disturbed. Take a deep breath and get comfortable.
2. Scrunch your toes and tighten your feet. Hold for 5–7 seconds, then exhale and release. Notice the difference between tension and relaxation.
3. Move up your body:
    - **Legs:** Tighten your calves and thighs, then release.
4. **Hips & stomach:** Squeeze your abdominal muscles, then let them soften.
    - **Shoulders & arms:** Shrug your shoulders up to your ears, then relax.
    - **Hands & face:** Make fists, scrunch your face, then release.
5. Scan for lingering tension and if any areas still feel tight, repeat the process.
6. End with full-body relaxation. Imagine a wave of relaxation washing over you from head to toe.

After you're done, pause for a moment and reflect:

- Which areas held the most tension?

- How does your body feel now compared to when you started?

Maybe you feel a little looser, a little more present. Maybe some spots still feel tight—that's okay. Awareness is the first step toward shifting your state, and now that you've tuned in, you can explore other ways to support your system.

Expanding Your Somatic Toolkit

Throughout this book, we've explored different ways to reconnect with your body and tune into its signals. Now, it's time to expand your toolkit with more ways to support regulation in your daily life. The good news? You have plenty of options.

- **Laughter:** A full-blown belly laugh or even a chuckle can work wonders for your nervous system. But what if laughter doesn't come easily? Here are a few ways to invite more of it into your life:
    - **Laughter exercises:** Yes, faking a laugh can actually trick your body into the real thing. Set aside a few minutes in a quiet space, take deep breaths, and start with exaggerated giggles or silent laughs. Stick with it—it might feel ridiculous at first, but your body will still release endorphins and melt away tension.
    - **Funny content on demand:** Actively seek out things that make you laugh. Follow content creators

who bring humor into your day, queue up a hilarious podcast, or swap that heavy drama for a feel-good sitcom. Laughter is contagious, even through a screen.
    - **Smile more:** Sounds too simple, but it works. Smiling—even if it starts as just muscle movement—can naturally shift your mood and make laughter more accessible. Try offering a smile to a stranger, your barista, or even your own reflection.
- **Social connection:** That sense of relief after a heart-to-heart with someone who gets you? That's your vagus nerve doing its thing. Warm interactions—a deep conversation, a shared laugh, or even just sitting with someone you trust—sends calming signals through your system, reinforcing feelings of safety and connection.
- **Tech-assisted support:** If you're curious about more direct methods, vagus nerve stimulation (VNS) is a growing field. These devices send gentle electrical pulses to engage vagal pathways and have been explored for stress management, trauma recovery, and even treatment-resistant conditions like depression and PTSD. While research is still unfolding, it's an intriguing option for those looking for additional support beyond self-led practices. If you want to dig deeper, resources like the Polyvagal Institute offer great insights.

Technology, movement, breathwork—these are all powerful tools for regulation. But there's one more piece of the puzzle that often gets overlooked: sound.

Your nervous system responds to vibration more than you might realize. The next section explores how sound and vibration can help bring your nervous system back to balance, often in ways you're already using without even realizing it. Let's take a closer look.

Using Sound and Vibration to Activate the Vagus Nerve

Sound has a way of cutting through the chaos—literally and figuratively. Whether it's the right song at the right time, the hum of your own voice, or the deep vibrations of a chant, sound is something your nervous system feels. Let's understand how the right kind of sound can be a direct line to regulate your nervous system.

Safe and Sound Protocol (SSP)

Imagine hearing a song that instantly wraps you in a warm, familiar hug—like your favorite throwback tune that transports you to a simpler time. That's the essence of the Safe and Sound Protocol (SSP). Developed by Dr. Stephen Porges, SSP is essentially a playlist for your nervous system that is carefully curated to gently guide your body from survival mode into a space where safety and connection become the norm (*Safe and Sound Protocol*, 2016).

Picture tuning into a radio where every note is softened, nostalgic, and oddly comforting. Those subtle shifts in tone and frequency work their magic by activating tiny muscles in your inner ear, sending reassuring signals straight to your vagus nerve. Users often describe feeling the vibrations in their muscles, a quiet nod from the body acknowledging the calm (Trauma Geek, 2023).

Led by a trained therapist, SSP sessions clock in at about five hours—not exactly a quick pit stop, but they pack a serious punch. Not ready to commit to the full ride? No worries. Dive into resources like the Polyvagal Institute to get a sneak peek at the magic.

Humming and Chanting

Now, let's talk about a tool you already have at your disposal: your voice. Your vocal cords are connected to your vagus nerve, making sound one of the simplest and most effective tools for nervous system regulation (Russell, 2022).

If you've ever chanted "OM" in a yoga class, you've unknowingly tapped into this effect. Those vibrations actively deactivate parts of the brain involved in detecting threats (like the amygdala) while promoting a deep sense of internal calm.

Exercise 56: The Hum Sound

Not a fan of chanting? No problem—humming works just as well. Whether it's a song you love or just a steady, low hum, the effect is the same: Vibrations travel through your throat, chest, and face, stimulating the vagus nerve and helping your system shift into a more regulated state.

Let's put it into practice:

1. Sit with a straight but relaxed posture, or stand with your feet evenly balanced.
2. Inhale through your nose and exhale through your mouth silently until your breathing feels steady and natural.
3. Inhale through your nose, then exhale while making a gentle "hmmm" sound with closed lips. Notice the vibrations on your lips.
4. Keep the hum at a comfortable pitch, avoiding strain. If you feel tension, pause and relax before continuing.
5. Repeat 10 times, letting the vibrations flow naturally.

Exercise 57: The Voo Sound

If that gentle hum leaves you wanting more, there's an alternative that takes relaxation even deeper: the "vooo" sound, recommended by Dr. Peter Levine (Ally, 2020). This long, drawn-out vibration moves deep through your body, offering a surprisingly potent sense of grounding.

. . .

Let's try it:

1. Sit comfortably with both feet resting on the floor. Close your eyes or keep a soft, downward gaze.
2. Simply observe your natural breathing without changing it yet.
3. Inhale slowly through your nose, expanding your belly. Check that your shoulders stay still—this ensures true belly breathing.
4. Exhale as you let out a deep, foghorn-like "voo" sound, stretching it for as long as is comfortable. Feel the vibrations in your chest, arms, and legs.
5. Repeat for 3–5 minutes, allowing each cycle to deepen your relaxation.
6. When you're ready, gently move your fingers or rotate your ankles, and then slowly open your eyes.

Now, time to reflect:

- Where did you feel the vibrations the most while humming or chanting? Did any areas feel particularly soothing or tense?

_____
_____
_____

- Did any memories, thoughts, or emotions come up during the exercises? If so, how did you respond to them?

_____
_____
_____

These practices remind us that healing is simple and accessible. The tools are already within you—it's just a matter of tuning in.

As we approach the end of this book, it's time to take everything we've explored in it and shape it into something you can carry forward. The next step is taking what you've learned and turning it into something that feels doable, safe, and like the beginning of a new way of being.

12

YOUR 28-DAY SOMATIC THERAPY PLAN

BEFORE YOU START THINKING this is the end of your journey, let's be real: healing isn't about reaching some perfect finish line. It's about building a relationship with your body that supports you every day, through the highs, the lows, and everything in between.

We've covered a lot in this book—how trauma and stress show up in the body, why the nervous system holds onto experiences, and, most importantly, how to work with your body to release, regulate, and restore balance. Now, it's time to put all of that into action with a 28-day somatic therapy plan.

And here's the best part—you only need 10 minutes a day to feel a difference. That's it. Just 10 minutes. Think about how often you give away 10 minutes without even realizing it—scrolling on your phone, stressing about things outside your control, or overthinking the day ahead. But what if you took those 10 minutes and gifted them to yourself instead? What if you used them to reconnect, to breathe, to release, and to reset?

These 10 minutes aren't just another task to check off your to-do list. They're a chance to remind yourself that you matter. That your body deserves care. That your nervous system, which has been working so hard to keep you safe, deserves moments of peace. Over time, these small daily practices will build resilience, increase emotional regulation, and help untangle the lingering effects of trauma and stress. Small moments of mindfulness and movement add up, rewiring your body's response to stress and creating a sense of safety from the inside out.

So, I want you to make yourself a promise. For the next 28 days, commit to these 10 minutes. Not because you *should*, but because you *deserve* it.

This plan isn't about doing things perfectly. Some days, you'll feel deeply connected to the exercises. Other days, you might struggle to engage. That's okay. The goal is to show up for yourself, even if it's just for a few moments. Think of this as a guided experiment—one that helps you discover what works best for your body and mind.

Best Tips for Using This 28-Day Plan

Before diving in, here are a few things to keep in mind:

1. **Listen to Your Body** – Some exercises might feel amazing; others might stir up emotions. That's normal. If something feels too much, adjust it or take a break.
2. **Create a Ritual** – Consistency is key. Whether it's morning, afternoon, or before bed, try to set a time each day for your somatic practice.
3. **Journal Your Experience** – Jot down sensations, thoughts, or emotions that come up. You might start noticing patterns over time.
4. **Be Gentle with Yourself** – Healing isn't linear. Some days will feel easier than others, and that's totally fine.
5. **Find What Works** – This plan is a starting point. If certain exercises really resonate with you, keep them in your routine even after the 28 days.

28-Day Somatic Therapy Plan

This 28-day somatic plan is all about tuning into your body, easing stress, and feeling more present in your daily life. Each day, you'll explore two simple exercises that build on each other. Some will feel like a perfect fit, others might surprise you, and that's all part of the process. There's no rush, no pressure—just an invitation to show up, explore, and see what works for you.

Day 1: Foundations of Self-Awareness

- **Exercise 1:** The Three Whys (Self-Reflection)
- **Exercise 2:** The Body Scan (Checking in With Your Body)
- **Why these exercises:** A strong start! We're setting the tone with self-reflection and checking in. Self-awareness is the first step to healing.

Day 2: Mindful Engagement

- **Exercise 1:** Mindful Walking (Awareness in Motion)
- **Exercise 2:** STOP Technique (Pause and Regulate)
- **Why these exercises:** Learning to stay present while moving through daily life makes mindfulness more accessible.

Day 3: Somatic Tracking for Safety

- **Exercise 1:** Somatic Tracking Meditation (Noticing Sensations)
- **Exercise 2:** Palm Pushing (Releasing Stored Tension)
- **Why these exercises:** We're noticing where we hold tension and actively releasing it. A powerful combo.

Day 4: Breath as a Tool

- **Exercise 1:** Diaphragmatic Breathing (Calming the Nervous System)
- **Exercise 2:** The Hum Sound (Vagal Nerve Stimulation)
- **Why these exercises:** Breathwork soothes the nervous system, and humming activates the vagus nerve for deeper relaxation.

Day 5: Connecting to the Present

- **Exercise 1:** Sit and Observe (Sensory Awareness)
- **Exercise 2:** Grounding With an Anchoring Statement (Emotional Stability)
- **Why these exercises:** Engaging the senses + grounding = a solid way to feel safe and stable.

Day 6: Emotional Regulation

- **Exercise 1:** Riding the Wave (Allowing Emotions to Flow)
- **Exercise 2:** Opposite Action (Rewiring Emotional Responses)
- **Why these exercises:** Learning to flow with emotions and shift responses instead of suppressing them.

Day 7: Reflection and Resourcing

- **Exercise 1:** Five-Step Resourcing (Building Inner Strength)
- **Exercise 2:** The Wheel of Awareness Meditation (Expanding Awareness)

- **Why these exercises:** Strengthening your internal resources makes stressful moments easier to handle.

Day 8: Releasing Physical Tension

- **Exercise 1:** 60-Second Somatic Tension Release (Quick Release)
- **Exercise 2:** Guided Imagery (Visualizing Calm)
- **Why these exercises:** One helps shake off tension fast, the other calms you through visualization.

Day 9: Grounding in Nature and Self-Touch

- **Exercise 1:** Nature Walk With Intention (Grounding in Nature)
- **Exercise 2:** The Gentle Hand Technique (Soothing Self-Touch)
- **Why these exercises:** Grounding outside and calming with gentle self-touch makes for a nourishing reset.

Day 10: Emotional Labeling and Awareness

- **Exercise 1:** Labeling and Categorizing Emotions (Naming What You Feel)
- **Exercise 2:** Breathe and Press (Grounding Through Pressure)
- **Why these exercises:** Brings clarity to emotional experience while using the body to stay grounded.

Day 11: Deep Sensory Awareness

- **Exercise 1:** Somatic Awareness and Tracking (Tuning into Sensations)

- **Exercise 2:** Sit and Observe (Sensory Awareness)
- **Why these exercises:** Refines your ability to track sensations while staying grounded and present.

Day 12: Emotional Resilience

- **Exercise 1:** EFT Tapping (Emotional Regulation)
- **Exercise 2:** Grounding with an Anchoring Statement (Emotional Stability)
- **Why these exercises:** Regulate and center yourself through tapping and intentional grounding phrases.

Day 13: Vagal Toning and Vocal Activation

- **Exercise 1:** The Voo Sound (Vagal Activation)
- **Exercise 2:** Somatic Sighing (Letting Go)
- **Why these exercises:** These vagal nerve techniques ease tension through vocal vibration and breath.

Day 14: Movement for Emotional Flow

- **Exercise 1:** Shake It Off (Stress Release)
- **Exercise 2:** Dance It Out (Expressive Movement)
- **Why these exercises:** Movement unlocks emotional expression and releases tension.

Day 15: Breath Variation and Control

- **Exercise 1:** The Double Inhale Method (Regulating with Breath)
- **Exercise 2:** Bilateral Stimulation (Left-Right Nervous System Balance)

- **Why these exercises:** These breath techniques support deeper nervous system regulation through intentional rhythms and bilateral activation.

Day 16: Releasing Tension Through Stretching

- **Exercise 1:** Neck Side Stretch (Upper Body Relief)
- **Exercise 2:** Supine Spinal Twist (Spinal Release)
- **Why these exercises:** Gentle upper body release combined with spinal movement to unwind deeply held tension.

Day 17: Massage-Based Reset

- **Exercise 1:** Neck and Shoulder Tension Release (Targeted Relief)
- **Exercise 2:** Full Body Relaxation with a Tool (Soothing Muscle Reset)
- **Why these exercises:** These massage techniques melt away muscle tightness and calm the entire system.

Day 18: Gentle Somatic Yoga

- **Exercise 1:** Reclined Pigeon Pose (Hip Release)
- **Exercise 2:** Seated Forward Bend Pose (Hamstring + Spine Stretch)
- **Why these exercises:** These help open up areas where stress settles, supporting mobility and calm.

Day 19: Qigong-Inspired Grounding

- **Exercise 1:** The Gathering Breath (Qigong Breathwork)
- **Exercise 2:** Swaying Tree (Qigong Movement)

- **Why these exercises:** These gentle flowing movements create rhythm and grounded energy in the body.

Day 20: Releasing Resistance

- **Exercise 1:** Pendulation and Titration (Balancing Activation)
- **Exercise 2:** Sequencing (Processing and Releasing)
- **Why these exercises:** These practices help let go of internal resistance and promote ease.

Day 21: Rebuilding Boundaries and Inner Strength

- **Exercise 1:** Exploring Boundaries with Hands (Physical Boundaries)
- **Exercise 2:** Toward and Away (Boundary Exploration)
- **Why these exercises:** Hands-on boundary work helps identify personal space and emotional comfort levels.

Day 22: Self-Support and Stability

- **Exercise 1:** Sit and Observe (Sensory Awareness)
- **Exercise 2:** How Can I Resource Myself? (Emotional Safety)
- **Why these exercises:** Build inner stability by noticing what's happening inside before it overwhelms you.

Day 23: Vagal Nerve Regulation

- **Exercise 1:** Tracking Your Nervous System (Monitoring Activation)
- **Exercise 2:** Expanding Your Window of Tolerance (Building Capacity)

- **Why these exercises:** Learn to notice your body's cues and stretch your tolerance gently over time.

Day 24: Deep Grounding and Support

- **Exercise 1:** Sole Connection (Grounding Through Feet)
- **Exercise 2:** Breathe and Press (Breath-Body Anchoring)
- **Why these exercises:** These exercises reinforce stability, helping you feel grounded, present, and supported.

Day 25: Integrating Movement and Breath

- **Exercise 1:** Bridge Pose (Hip and Spine Opener)
- **Exercise 2:** Cat-Cow Pose (Spinal Flexibility)
- **Why these exercises:** Movement-based somatic work creates flexibility in both the body and nervous system.

Day 26: Self-Compassion and Healing

- **Exercise 1:** The Gentle Hand Technique (Nurturing Touch)
- **Exercise 2:** Progressive Muscle Relaxation (Full-Body Unwinding)
- **Why these exercises:** Combining gentle touch with full-body relaxation fosters deep self-kindness.

Day 27: Nervous System Closure

- **Exercise 1:** The 2-Step Self-Holding Exercise (Comforting Touch)
- **Exercise 2:** Somatic Breath Counting (Breath Awareness)

- **Why these exercises:** Close out the journey with gentle touch and breath—simple tools you can always return to.

Day 28: Reflection and Looking Ahead

- **Exercise 1:** Daily Journaling (Reflective Journaling)
- **Exercise 2:** The Wheel of Awareness Meditation (Expanding Awareness)
- **Why these exercises:** Wrapping it up with reflection and considering how to integrate these tools long-term.

As you implement these exercises into your day, some exercises may stick with you, while others might not feel like your thing—and that's totally okay. The real takeaway is knowing you have tools to support yourself whenever you need them. Keep practicing what feels good, stay curious, and remember—your body is always on your side.

Making Somatics Work for You

You've built a great toolkit of somatic practices to help you reconnect and feel at home in your body. But knowing what to do and actually doing it? Two very different things. Stress doesn't care if you have a self-care plan. It shows up uninvited, usually at the worst possible moment. You wake up tense. A conversation drains you. Your body reacts before your brain even catches up. So, how do you make these practices part of your actual day instead of something you forget about until you're overwhelmed?

By now, you might've started slipping some of these practices into your day—maybe a breath here, a stretch there. Small shifts add up, but as we near the end of this journey, let's make sure your toolkit stays stocked with options. Let's dive in.

Morning: Waking Up in a Way That Supports Your Nervous System

As soon as you open your eyes, your body's already plotting its day—so why not give it a friendly nudge in the right direction? If you've got a leisurely start, try the Sole Connection exercise: Feel those feet connect with the floor like you're grounding yourself for greatness. Mix in a few rounds of Diaphragmatic Breathing or the Double Inhale Method to gently wake up your system. If you're in mad dash mode, don't fret—a quick round of Shake It Off can help jolt you awake without any fuss. These exercises are like your morning espresso for the nervous system. They set you up to handle whatever the day throws your way.

During the Day: Staying Present, Connected, and Balanced

When you're in the thick of it—stuck at your desk or running errands—well-timed exercises can make a real difference. If you're waiting for the elevator, try The Elevator Breather to keep calm and carry on. Caught in traffic? The Traffic Light Breath is your new best friend—sync your breathing with those red lights and enjoy the mini-break. And if you're on the move, The Walking Breath is a great way to keep your rhythm in check. These little practices are quick, smart, and just the right amount of playful to help you stay balanced in the hustle.

Evening: Releasing the Day and Resetting Before Sleep

As the evening settles in, it's time to let go of the day's momentum and give your nervous system a gentle goodnight kiss. If you're still carrying a bit of tension, the Rock-and-Breathe Hug or the comforting 2-step Self-holding Exercise can be just the trick to say, "Hey, it's okay—I've got you." For those nights when your mind's buzzing like a busy café, try Journaling in Small Doses; just a few words can help unload your thoughts. If you'd prefer a more physical approach, a short session of Somatic Tracking Meditation allows you to check in with your body before bed. Finally, The Hum or The Voo Sound can help your system wind down, signaling that it's time to rest and recharge.

When Old Trauma Responses Sneak In

We all have those moments when past storms resurface uninvited. When that happens, think of your exercises as a trusty toolkit. Start with The Three Whys—ask "why" three times to peel back those layers and get to the heart of what's really going on. Let yourself Ride the Wave, allowing emotions to rise and fall without judgment. If you're tempted to retreat, why not experiment with Opposite Action and gently nudge yourself toward a different response? If you're still feeling off-balance, a dash of Pendulation can shift your focus between discomfort and a neutral zone.

In Chapter 8, you tried the Pendulation *and* Titration exercise, to help you explore these methods at your own pace. If you'd like more support, consider scheduling one or two sessions per week with a somatic therapist. Professional guidance can make all the difference in how quickly (and comfortably) you learn to pendulate between challenging sensations and your resources. After practicing in a safe, supported environment, you'll be better able to decide how much of these techniques to integrate into your everyday life based on your own comfort level and progress.

That shift—moving from reacting to responding, from feeling stuck to discovering choice—is the heart of somatic work. It's building a foundation where your nervous system can recover faster, where moments of regulation come more easily, and where you trust your body's ability to find its way back to balance.

This evolution mirrors a broader change in how we approach healing. For decades, mental health centered on talk therapies that dissected thoughts and beliefs. Today, research shows that our bodies play a vital role in recovery, with somatic practices now key in trauma therapy, chronic pain management, and even workplace wellness.

Breathwork, movement, and nervous system regulation have shifted from the margins to essential tools for well-being. Meanwhile, cutting-edge technologies—from wearable devices that measure stress responses in real-time to virtual reality programs that offer immersive experiences for self-regulation—are expanding how we engage with healing. The future of somatic therapy is unfolding before our eyes, bridging the mind-body gap with unprecedented clarity and impact.

The field is evolving, but one thing stays the same: Your body holds wisdom. And now, you know how to listen.

Moving Forward with Somatic Practices

So, where do you go from here? The short answer: wherever feels right for you.

This plan isn't something you complete and then forget about. It's a roadmap—a collection of tools you can return to whenever you need them. Maybe you'll continue cycling through these exercises, or maybe you'll find a few favorites to weave into your daily routine. Either way, you now have the foundation to support yourself in moments of stress, overwhelm, or uncertainty.

Remember, healing isn't about fixing yourself—it's about learning to work with yourself. At times, it might look like deep breathing and movement; at other moments, it could be as simple as placing a hand on your heart and taking a moment to pause.

Your body has always been on your side. Now, you have the tools to listen, trust, and respond in a way that nurtures and heals.

You've got this. And when in doubt? Just take one deep breath at a time.

CONCLUSION

Just like that, here we are—the last page, the final stretch. If this book were a yoga class, this would be *Savasana*: that moment when you're lying still, your body heavy, and your mind finally quiets down instead of rehashing that awkward thing you said two weeks ago.

Really take a second. You made it here—page by page, breath by breath, step by step. That's no small thing.

Along the way, you've learned that your body isn't just a warehouse of tension or a record of old hurts; it's a living, breathing guide, capable of release and renewal. When your jaw relaxed for the first time, maybe you felt a door crack open, like an invitation to listen more closely. Then, when you took a few conscious breaths in a stressful moment, you witnessed how quickly your entire mood could shift. In those moments, you began to realize that healing isn't an overnight process or a race toward perfection; it's an ongoing journey back to yourself.

With that in mind, I want you to remember there might still be days when tension drops by, or your mind replays old worries on endless repeat. That doesn't mean you've failed. It simply means you're alive. Life can test us, but now you have tools—simple, powerful ways to anchor yourself. You know how to pause. You know how to listen. You know that your body is working with you.

So, where do you go from here?

You start where you are. Maybe that means choosing one practice that felt good and making it part of your routine. A body scan before bed, a moment to check in with your breath before the day starts, or getting used to leaning on your resources when you need to feel stable and safe. Or, perhaps, it means sharing what you've learned with someone who needs it. Whatever it looks like, the important thing is that you keep going. Keep trusting in your body's ability to shift, to release, to heal. It's been waiting for you to listen all along.

If you ever feel like you need extra support, know that you don't have to do this alone. There are resources—books, workshops, therapists, communities—people who understand and can walk this path with you.

Your body is wise. Your nervous system is resilient. And you? You are capable of so much more than you think.

So, take a breath. Feel your heartbeat. Let that steady rhythm remind you:

I am here. I am listening. I am healing.

That's everything.

CONCLUSION

Keeping the Word Alive

Now you have everything you need to regulate your nervous system, relieve stress, and strengthen your mind-body connection, it's time to pass on your newfound knowledge and show other readers where they can find the same help.

Simply by leaving your honest opinion of this book on Amazon, you'll show other readers curious about somatic therapy where they can find the information they're looking for and pass their passion for healing forward.

Thank you for your help. Somatic therapy is kept alive when we pass on our knowledge – and you're helping me to do just that.

To make a difference, simply scan the QR code and leave a review: https://www.amazon.com/review/review-your-purchases/?asin=1764076109

BIBLIOGRAPHY

Ackerman, C. E. (2018, February 5). *21 emotion regulation worksheets & strategies*. Positive Psychology. https://positivepsychology.com/emotion-regulation-worksheets-strategies-dbt-skills/

Agorastos, A., & Olff, M. (2020). Traumatic stress and the circadian system: Neurobiology, timing and treatment of posttraumatic chronodisruption. *European Journal of Psychotraumatology, 11*(1), 1833644. https://doi.org/10.1080/20008198.2020.1833644

Alexander technique. (2020). NHS. https://www.nhs.uk/conditions/alexander-technique/

Allen, Dr. S. (2018, April 27). *7 simple grounding techniques for calming down quickly*. Dr. Sarah Allen Counseling. https://drsarahallen.com/7-ways-to-calm/

Ally, C. (2020, February 11). *Trauma care VOO breathing*. Flourish Counseling Co. https://flourishcounseling.co/trauma-care-voo-breathing/

Asmundson, G. J. G., Fetzner, M. G., DeBoer, L. B., Powers, M. B., Otto, M. W., & Smits, J. A. J. (2013). Let's get physical: A contemporary review of the anxiolytic effects of exercise for anxiety and its disorders. *Depression and Anxiety, 30*(4), 362–373. https://doi.org/10.1002/da.22043

Aziz-Zadeh, L., & Damasio, A. (2008). Embodied semantics for actions: Findings from functional brain imaging. *Journal of Physiology-Paris, 102*(1-3), 35–39. https://doi.org/10.1016/j.jphysparis.2008.03.012

Berger, M. W. (2021, January 6). *Self-awareness can drive behavior change, reprogram the brain's reward system*. Penn Today. https://penntoday.upenn.edu/news/Penn-research-self-awareness-behavior-change-reprogram-brain-reward-system

Bioenergetic therapy by alexander lowen: Principles and benefits - mentesabiertaspsicologia.com. (2023, February). Mentes Abiertas Psicología. https://www.mentesabiertaspsicologia.com/blog-psicologia/bioenergetic-therapy-by-alexander-lowen-principles-and-benefits#google_vignette

Blankenship, B. (2023, November). *Exercises and examples of somatic experiencing therapy*. Balanced Awakening, P.C. https://balancedawakening.com/blog/exercises-and-examples-of-somatic-experiencing-therapy

Boadella, D. (1974). *Wilhelm Reich: the evolution of his work*. Internet Archive. https://archive.org/details/wilhelmreichevol0000boad

Bremner, J. D. (2006). Traumatic stress: Effects on the brain. *Dialogues in Clinical Neuroscience, 8*(4), 445–461. https://doi.org/10.31887/dcns.2006.8.4/jbremner

Brenner, B. (2024, March 14). *The essential guide to somatic therapy: Navigating mind-body healing*. Therapy Group of NYC. https://nyctherapy.com/therapists-nyc-blog/the-essential-guide-to-somatic-therapy-navigating-mind-body-healing/

Brom, D., Stokar, Y., Lawi, C., Nuriel-Porat, V., Ziv, Y., Lerner, K., & Ross, G. (2017).

Somatic experiencing for posttraumatic stress disorder: A randomized controlled outcome study. *Journal of Traumatic Stress, 30*(3), 304–312. https://doi.org/10.1002/jts.22189

Brown, L., Rando, A. A., Eichel, K., Van Dam, N. T., Celano, C. M., Huffman, J. C., & Morris, M. E. (2020). The effects of mindfulness and meditation on vagally-mediated heart rate variability. *Psychosomatic Medicine, Publish Ahead of Print.* https://doi.org/10.1097/psy.0000000000000900

Brown, R. P., & Gerbarg, P. L. (2005). Sudarshan kriya yogic breathing in the treatment of stress, anxiety, and depression: Part i—neurophysiologic model. *The Journal of Alternative and Complementary Medicine, 11*(1), 189–201. https://doi.org/10.1089/acm.2005.11.189

Carefoot, H. (2023, August 17). *I'm a trauma-informed somatic practitioner, and here's how to use somatic boundaries to protect your mental health.* Well+Good. https://www.wellandgood.com/somatic-boundaries/

Carney, D. R., Cuddy, A. J. C., & Yap, A. J. (2010). Power posing: Brief nonverbal displays affect neuroendocrine levels and risk tolerance. *Psychological Science, 21*(10), 1363–1368. https://doi.org/10.1177/0956797610383437

Cellarius, P. (2023, August 23). *The remarkable benefits of somatic experiencing.* GoodTherapy. https://www.goodtherapy.org/blog/benefits-of-somatic-experiencing/

Center for Substance Abuse Treatment. (2014). *Understanding the impact of trauma.* National Library of Medicine; Substance Abuse and Mental Health Services Administration (US). https://www.ncbi.nlm.nih.gov/books/NBK207191/

Cherry, K. (2024, July 14). *The 6 types of basic emotions and their effect on human behavior.* Verywell Mind. https://www.verywellmind.com/an-overview-of-the-types-of-emotions-4163976

Choi, A. (2024, July 3). *What is somatic mindfulness and qigong?* Brainz Magazine. https://www.brainzmagazine.com/post/what-is-somatic-mindfulness-and-qigong

Chopra, D. (2024). *Deepak Chopra quote.* Quotefancy. https://quotefancy.com/quote/792552/Deepak-Chopra-The-mind-and-the-body-are-like-parallel-universes-Anything-that-happens-in

Clarke, J. (2019). *Polyvagal theory and how it relates to social cues.* Verywell Mind. https://www.verywellmind.com/polyvagal-theory-4588049

Clear, J. (2018). *Atomic habits: Tiny changes, remarkable results.* Avery, An Imprint Of Penguin Random House. https://dn790007.ca.archive.org/0/items/atomic-habits-pdfdrive/Atomic%20habits%20%28%20PDFDrive%20%29.pdf

Davis, I., Rovers, M., & Petrella, C. (2017). Touch deprivation and counselling as healing touch. *Touch in the Helping Professions,* 13–32. https://doi.org/10.2307/j.ctv5vdcvd.5

A deeper look into how and why EFT is so effective. (2015). Tapping Works. https://www.tappingworks.co.uk/how-eft-works

de Kamp, M. M., Scheffers, M., Hatzmann, J., Emck, C., Cuijpers, P., & Beek, P. J. (2019). Body- and movement-oriented interventions for posttraumatic stress disorder: A systematic review and meta-analysis. *Journal of Traumatic Stress, 32*(6), 967–976. https://doi.org/10.1002/jts.22465

de Ridder, D. T. D., Lensvelt-Mulders, G., Finkenauer, C., Stok, F. M., & Baumeister, R. F. (2012). Taking stock of self-control: A meta-analysis of how trait self-control relates to a wide range of behaviors. *Personality and Social Psychology Review: An Official Journal of the Society for Personality and Social Psychology, Inc, 16*(1), 76–99. https://doi.org/10.1177/1088868311418749

Dr. Stephen Porges' Safe and Sound Protocol. (n.d.). Unyte Integrated Listening. https://integratedlistening.com/polyvagal-theory/porges/

Dubois-Maahs, J. (2020, October 16). *What is somatic therapy and how can it benefit you?* Talkspace. https://www.talkspace.com/blog/somatic-therapy-what-is-definition-get-started-guide/

Egberts, J. (2023, May 4). *Exploring the origins and history of breathwork.* Breathless. https://breathlessexpeditions.com/origins-history-of-breathwork/

Elbrecht, C. (2022, October 22). *Pendulation as a core trauma healing model.* Institute for Sensorimotor Art Therapy. https://www.sensorimotorarttherapy.com/blog/pendulation-as-a-core-trauma-healing-model

Emma, & Carla. (2024, March 6). *37 mind body connection quotes for inner peace.* Merrymaker Sisters. https://themerrymakersisters.com/mind-body-connection-quotes/

Exercise 4: Supportive Touch. (n.d.). Self-Compassion. https://self-compassion.org/exercises/exercise-4-supportive-touch/

Exploring somatic experiencing exercises for self-care. (2024, April 15). Talk. Heal. Thrive. https://talkhealthrive.com/post/exploring-somatic-experiencing-exercises-for-self-care/

Exploring the evidence behind somatic therapy: Is it truly effective? (2023, October 24). Inspire Malibu. https://www.inspiremalibu.com/blog/mental-health/evidence-behind-somatic-therapy-is-it-truly-effective/

Folk, J. (2022, April 25). *Anxiety buzzing sensations.* AnxietyCentre.com. https://www.anxietycentre.com/anxiety-disorders/symptoms/buzzing-sensations/

Forman, B. (2024, May 30). *How does trauma impact the immune system?* Immunology & Microbiology from Technology Networks; Technology Networks. https://www.technologynetworks.com/immunology/news/how-does-trauma-impact-the-immune-system-387261

Forte, T. (2019, October 22). *The body keeps the score: Brain, mind, and body in the treatment of trauma (book summary).* Forte Labs. https://fortelabs.com/blog/the-body-keeps-the-score-summary/

Gauci Bongiovanni, M. (2023, September 11). *What is somatic tracking for chronic pain?* PainOutsideTheBox. https://www.painoutsidethebox.com/tms-blog/somatic-tracking

González-Ramírez, M. L., García-Vázquez, J. P., Rodríguez, M. D., Padilla-López, L. A., Galindo-Aldana, G., & Cuevas-González, D. (2023). Wearables for Stress Management: A Scoping Review. *Healthcare, 11*(17), 2369–2369. https://doi.org/10.3390/healthcare11172369

Gordan, R., Gwathmey, J. K., & Xie, L.-H. (2015). Autonomic and endocrine control of cardiovascular function. *World Journal of Cardiology, 7*(4), 204–214. https://doi.org/10.4330/wjc.v7.i4.204

Grounding & Breathing Exercises for Calming Your Nervous System. (n.d.). Counseling & Psych Services. https://caps.arizona.edu/grounding

Gushée, S. R. (2017, January 13). *Sounds of my nightly routine: Chaos, singing, humming, and chanting om*. Medium. https://medium.com/thrive-global/sounds-of-my-nightly-routine-chaos-singing-humming-and-chanting-om-12a24e4c0b56

Hampton, C. (2023). *The Somatic Therapy Handbook:* Self-Soothing Techniques for Healing Trauma, Enhancing the Mind-Body Connection, and Stress Relief

Hampton, Cher. The Somatic Therapy Handbook: Self-Soothing Techniques for Healing Trauma, Enhancing the Mind-Body Connection, and Stress Relief (Holistic Health) (English Edition) . Independent. Edición de Kindle.

Hanna, T. (2016). *What is Somatics?* Somatic Systems Institute. https://somatics.org/library/htl-wis1

Hanshans, C., Tatjana Amler, Zauner, J., & Lukas Bröll. (2023). Inducing and measuring acute stress in virtual reality: Evaluation of canonical physiological stress markers and measuring methods. *Journal of Environmental Psychology*, 102107–102107. https://doi.org/10.1016/j.jenvp.2023.102107

Hanson, H. (n.d.). *Peter Levine 2-step holding exercise*. The art of healing trauma blog. https://www.new-synapse.com/aps/wordpress/wp-content/uploads/2016/04/printable-2-step-self-holding.pdf

History of breathwork. (n.d.). Mana Breathwork. https://manabreathwork.com/history-of-breathwork

Hofmann, S. G., Sawyer, A. T., Witt, A. A., & Oh, D. (2010). The effect of mindfulness-based therapy on anxiety and depression: A meta-analytic review. *Journal of Consulting and Clinical Psychology, 78*(2), 169–183. https://doi.org/10.1037/a0018555

Hum for your health: Why humming is so healing & how to do it. (n.d.). Flowly. https://www.flowly.world/post/hum-for-your-health-why-humming-is-so-healing-how-to-do-it

Humming exercises. (n.d.). Cambridge University Hospitals. https://www.cuh.nhs.uk/patient-information/humming-exercises/

Integrating somatic practices into everyday life. (2023, August 16). Repose. https://byrepose.com/journal/integrating-somatic-practices-into-everyday-life

Is Somatic Psychotherapy Right For You? (2021, April 16). Integrative Psychotherapy. https://integrativepsych.co/new-blog/is-somatic-therapy-right-for-you

Karadag, P., & Gillett, J. (2021). *Somatic practice and chronic pain*. Warwick. https://warwick.ac.uk/fac/sci/psych/research/lifespan/sleeplab/projects/within/blog/january2021/

Keng, S. L., Smoski, M. J., & Robins, C. J. (2011). Effects of mindfulness on psychological health: A review of empirical studies. *Clinical Psychology Review, 31*(6), 1041–1056. https://doi.org/10.1016/j.cpr.2011.04.006

Kilian, R., & LearnWellBooks. (2024). *Somatic exercises for nervous system regulation:*

35 beginner – intermediate techniques to reduce anxiety & tone your vagus nerve in under 10 minutes A day.

Kimble, S. (2023, March 24). *Movement heals all wounds.* Trauma Research Foundation. https://traumaresearchfoundation.org/movement-heals-all-wounds/

Klein, C. (2024). *Using virtual reality to support social and emotional learning.* NEA. https://www.nea.org/professional-excellence/student-engagement/tools-tips/using-virtual-reality-support-social-and-emotional-learning

Komariah, M., Ibrahim, K., Pahria, T., Rahayuwati, L., & Somantri, I. (2023). Effect of mindfulness breathing meditation on depression, anxiety, and stress: A randomized controlled trial among university students. *Healthcare, 11*(1), 26. https://doi.org/10.3390/healthcare11010026

König, N., Steber, S., Seebacher, J., von Prittwitz, Q., Bliem, H. R., & Rossi, S. (2019). How Therapeutic Tapping Can Alter Neural Correlates of Emotional Prosody Processing in Anxiety. *Brain Sciences, 9*(8). https://doi.org/10.3390/brainsci9080206

Kuhfuß, M., Maldei, T., Hetmanek, A., & Baumann, N. (2021). Somatic experiencing – effectiveness and key factors of a body-oriented trauma therapy: A scoping literature review. *European Journal of Psychotraumatology, 12*(1), 1–17. https://doi.org/10.1080/20008198.2021.1929023

Laborde, S., Mosley, E., & Thayer, J. F. (2017). Heart rate variability and cardiac vagal tone in psychophysiological research – recommendations for experiment planning, data analysis, and data reporting. *Frontiers in Psychology, 08*(213). https://doi.org/10.3389/fpsyg.2017.00213

Laderer, A. (2024, January 19). *5 vagus nerve exercises to help you chill out.* Charlie Health. https://www.charliehealth.com/post/vagus-nerve-exercises

Leary, M. R. (2015). Emotional responses to interpersonal rejection. *Emotions, 17*(4), 435–441. https://doi.org/10.31887/dcns.2015.17.4/mleary

Lebow, H. (2022, September 14). *How does your body remember trauma? Plus 5 ways to heal.* Psych Central. https://psychcentral.com/health/how-your-body-remembers-trauma#trauma-and-the-body

Leclercq, S., Forsythe, P., & Bienenstock, J. (2016). Posttraumatic stress disorder: Does the gut microbiome hold the key? *The Canadian Journal of Psychiatry, 61*(4), 204–213. https://doi.org/10.1177/0706743716635535

Lee, S., Kim, J. H., & Chung, J. H. (2021). The association between sleep quality and quality of life: A population-based study. *Sleep Medicine, 84,* 121–126. https://doi.org/10.1016/j.sleep.2021.05.022

Lemaistre, C. (n.d.). *HOMEBODY somatic grounding exercises for coming home to your body.* https://static1.squarespace.com/static/5940b47e5016e1c79e44370a/t/601b880d701b1b2da698c106/1612417038306/Home_Body+EBOOK.pdf

Levine, P. A. (n.d.). *Peter A. Levine quotes.* BrainyQuote. https://www.brainyquote.com/quotes/peter_a_levine_864302

Levine, P. A. (2014, March 17). *Dr. Peter Levine on the future of the Somatic Experiencing Approach.* PsychAlive. https://www.psychalive.org/video-dr-peter-levine-future-of-somatic-experiencing-approach/

Lowndes, C. (2021, August 25). *A brief history of somatic education*. Essential Somatics. https://essentialsomatics.com/a-brief-history-of-somatic-education/

Lozovyi, Y. (2023). *Somatic therapy workbook exercises to treat trauma, complex PTSD and dissociation: Mindfulness, self-compassion, and the mind-body approach to reduce stress and heal trauma*. Fiola Publishing.

Lumley, M. A., Cohen, J. L., Borszcz, G. S., Cano, A., Radcliffe, A. M., Porter, L. S., Schubiner, H., & Keefe, F. J. (2011). Pain and emotion: A biopsychosocial review of recent research. *Journal of Clinical Psychology, 67*(9), 942–968. https://doi.org/10.1002/jclp.20816

Lundberg, A. (2023, May 3). *How does your body remember trauma?* Charlie Health. https://www.charliehealth.com/post/how-does-your-body-remember-trauma

MA, C. E. A. (2018, July 3). *What is self-regulation? (+95 skills and strategies)*. PositivePsychology.com. https://positivepsychology.com/self-regulation/#adults-self-regulation

Ma, X., Yue, Z.-Q., Gong, Z.-Q., Zhang, H., Duan, N.-Y., Shi, Y.-T., Wei, G.-X., & Li, Y.-F. (2017). The effect of diaphragmatic breathing on attention, negative affect and stress in healthy adults. *Frontiers in Psychology, 8*(874), 1–12. https://doi.org/10.3389/fpsyg.2017.00874

Ma, Y., & Liu, Z. (2024). Emotion regulation and well-being as factors contributing to lessening burnout among Chinese EFL teachers. *Acta Psychologica, 245*, 104219. https://doi.org/10.1016/j.actpsy.2024.104219

Mahindru, A., Patil, P., & Agrawal, V. (2023). Role of physical activity on mental health and well-being: A review. *Cureus, 15*(1). https://doi.org/10.7759/cureus.33475

Making somatics part of your routine - part 2. (2020, November 20). Learn Somatics. https://learnsomatics.ie/making-somatics-part-of-your-routine-part-2/

Making somatics part of your routine - part 3. (2021, January 13). Learn Somatics. https://learnsomatics.ie/making-somatics-part-of-your-routine-part-3/

Making somatics part of your routine - part 4. (2021, January 13). Learn Somatics. https://learnsomatics.ie/making-somatics-part-of-your-routine-part-4/

Making somatics part of your routine – part 1. (2020, November 13). Learn Somatics. https://learnsomatics.ie/making-somatics-part-of-your-routine-part-1/

McCollum, S. (2019, September 5). *Your brain on music: The sound system between your ears*. The Kennedy Center. https://www.kennedy-center.org/education/resources-for-educators/classroom-resources/media-and-interactives/media/music/your-brain-on-music/your-brain-on-music/your-brain-on-music-the-sound-system-between-your-ears/

McLean, R. (2024, May 18). *Making sounds: "The Voo Sound"*. Medium. https://mcleanonline.medium.com/making-sounds-the-voo-sound-43e363b3826b

Meehan, E., & Carter, B. (2021). Moving with pain: What principles from somatic practices can offer to people living with chronic pain. *Frontiers in Psychology, 11*. https://doi.org/10.3389/fpsyg.2020.620381

Meletta, C. (2024, May 4). *Integrating somatic practices into everyday life to combat depression*. Courtnay Meletta. https://www.courtnaymeletta.com/post/integrating-somatic-practices-into-everyday-life-to-combat-depression

Michaels, K. (2023). *Becoming the body: Embodiment through somatic therapy.*

Migala, J. (2023, December 27). *How to stimulate your vagus nerve and why it matters.* EverydayHealth.com. https://www.everydayhealth.com/neurology/ways-to-stimulate-your-vagus-nerve-and-why-it-matters/

Millette, D. (2024, November 5). *6 steps to incorporate somatic therapy into your morning routine.* Brainz Magazine. https://www.brainzmagazine.com/post/6-steps-to-incorporate-somatic-therapy-into-your-morning-routine

Mind-body connection. (2025). Zencare. https://zencare.co/mental-health/mind-body-connection

Mischke-Reeds, M. (2018). *Somatic Psychotherapy Toolbox: 125 Worksheets and Exercises to Treat Trauma & Stress.* Pesi Publishing. https://static1.squarespace.com/static/5a1c1ef6cd39c36713a188df/t/64258d1a4e92ad5c09cd5689/1680182577863/Somatic-psychotherapy+toolbox++2.pdf

Mravec, B. (2006). Neurobiology of the stress response. *Shock, 25*(3), 315. https://doi.org/10.1097/01.shk.0000194031.31418.d5

Neacsiu, A. D., Rompogren, J., Eberle, J. W., & McMahon, K. (2018). Changes in problematic anger, shame, and disgust in anxious and depressed adults undergoing treatment for emotion dysregulation. *Behavior Therapy, 49*(3), 344–359. https://doi.org/10.1016/j.beth.2017.10.004

Nichols, A. (2024, March 7). *When healing gets handsy.* ELLE. https://www.elle.com/beauty/health-fitness/a60083026/what-is-somatic-therapy/

Norbury, J. W., Guo, Y., Boyer, P. J., & Zeri, R. S. (2018). The power of doppler in the popliteal fossa: Sonographic diagnosis of a fibular nerve neurofibroma in a patient with posterior knee swelling. *American Journal of Physical Medicine & Rehabilitation, 97*(10), e100–e101. https://doi.org/10.1097/phm.0000000000000928

Noyed, D. (2023, May 15). *Weighted blanket benefits.* Sleep Foundation. https://www.sleepfoundation.org/best-weighted-blankets/weighted-blanket-benefits

Orit Krug . (2020, June 19). *How dance therapy releases trauma from the nervous system.* Orit Krug | Dance Movement Therapist. https://oritkrug.com/how-dance-therapy-releases-trauma/

Örün, D., Karaca, S., & Arıkan, Ş. (2021). The effect of breathing exercise on stress hormones. *Cyprus Journal of Medical Sciences, 6*(1), 22–27. https://doi.org/10.4274/cjms.2021.2020.2390

Pascoe, M. C., Thompson, D. R., Jenkins, Z. M., & Ski, C. F. (2017). Mindfulness mediates the physiological markers of stress: Systematic review and meta-analysis. *Journal of Psychiatric Research, 95,* 156–178. https://doi.org/10.1016/j.jpsychires.2017.08.004

Paturel, A. (2024, March 21). *Bolster your brain by stimulating the vagus nerve.* Cedars-Sinai. https://www.cedars-sinai.org/blog/stimulating-the-vagus-nerve.html

Perelmuter, T. (2023, May 9). *What's the deal with humming meditation? Pros and cons.* EastWesticism. https://www.eastwesticism.org/humming-meditation/

Pietrangelo, A. (2023, March 21). *The effects of stress on your body.* Healthline. https://www.healthline.com/health/stress/effects-on-body

Porges, S. W. (2022). *The polyvagal theory: Neurophysiological foundations of emotions, attachment, communication, and self-regulation.* Internet Archive. https://archive.org/details/polyvagaltheoryn0000porg

The power of somatic healing. (2023, November 2). Integrated Spine, Pain & Wellness. https://ispwscottsdale.com/the-power-of-somatic-healing/

Quinn, D. (2023, May 25). *Somatic therapy: Understanding the mind-body connection.* Sandstone Care. https://www.sandstonecare.com/blog/somatic-therapy/

Rachel. (2024, August 6). *Somatic grounding exercises for self-regulation.* Yoga with Rachel. https://www.yogawithrachelmarie.com/post/somatic-grounding-exercises#viewer-0z7571086

Ramirez-Duran, D. (2020, November 11). *Somatic experiencing: Healing trauma with body-mind therapy.* PositivePsychology.com. https://positivepsychology.com/somatic-experiencing/

Raypole, C. (2019, May 24). *Grounding techniques: 30 techniques for anxiety, PTSD, and more.* Healthline. https://www.healthline.com/health/grounding-techniques#mental-techniques

Raypole, C. (2020, April 17). *Somatics: Definition, exercises, evidence, and more.* Healthline. https://www.healthline.com/health/somatics#does-it-work

Riaz, A., & Akuretiya, S. (2023, November 23). *Somatic dance: Liberation through expression and movement.* BetterMe Blog. https://betterme.world/articles/somatic-dance/

Rigby, A. (2024). *12 emotional regulation skills to calm your inner chaos.* Marlee. https://getmarlee.com/blog/emotional-regulation-skills

Rush, T., & Leonard, J. (2019, September 26). *What is EFT tapping? Evidence and how-to guide.* Medical News Today. https://www.medicalnewstoday.com/articles/326434

Russell, N. (2022, November 26). *Voice, the vagus nerve and co-regulation: Could they be one solution when supporting children?* LinkedIn. https://www.linkedin.com/pulse/voice-vagus-nerve-co-regulation-could-one-solution-when-nic-russell/

Safe and sound protocol: A portal to social engagement. (2016, December). Integrated Listening Australia. https://integratedlistening.com.au/ssp-safe-sound-protocol/

The science of hugs: Unraveling the power of physical touch. (2023, November 28). Positive Reset Mental Health Services of Eatontown New Jersey. https://positivereseteatontown.com/the-science-of-hugs-unraveling-the-power-of-physical-touch/

SE 101. (n.d.). Somatic Experiencing International. https://traumahealing.org/se-101/

SEI Communications. (2024, January 29). *SEI Connections Origins Story.* Somatic Experiencing® International. https://traumahealing.org/sei-connections-origins-story/

Sheard, R., & Davidson, A. (2023). Sustained practice of qigong results in a somatic hermeneutic process, contributing to appreciation of life. an interpretative phenomenological analysis. *Journal of Bodywork and Movement Therapies, 36,* 100–108. https://doi.org/10.1016/j.jbmt.2023.06.002

Sherman, K. J., Ludman, E. J., Cook, A. J., Hawkes, R. J., Roy-Byrne, P. P., Bentley, S., Brooks, M. Z., & Cherkin, D. C. (2010). Effectiveness of therapeutic massage for generalized anxiety disorder: A randomized controlled trial. *Depression and Anxiety, 27*(5), 441–450. https://doi.org/10.1002/da.20671

Siegel, D. (n.d.). *Wheel of awareness.* Dr. Dan Siegel. https://drdansiegel.com/wheel-of-awareness/

Siegel, D. (2018, August 21). *Dr. Dan Siegel's wheel of awareness.* Garrison Institute. https://www.garrisoninstitute.org/the-wheel-of-awareness/

Somatic tracking exercise. (n.d.). BCH Center for Mind Body Medicine. Retrieved January 25, 2025, from https://www.bch.org/documents/content/somatic-tracking-exercise.pdf

Starling, J. (2024). *Somatic Therapy for the Mind-Body Connection: A Beginners Guide to Healing Trauma and Relieving Chronic Stress and Tension With Easy "On-The-Go" Psychosomatic Exercises.*

Stress effects on the body. (2018, November 1). American Psychological Association. https://www.apa.org/topics/stress/body

Suzuki, M., Jagger, A. L., Konya, C., Shimojima, Y., Pryshchep, S., Goronzy, J. J., & Weyand, C. M. (2012). CD8+CD45RA+CCR7+FOXP3+ T cells with immunosuppressive properties: A novel subset of inducible human regulatory T cells. *The Journal of Immunology, 189*(5), 2118–2130. https://doi.org/10.4049/jimmunol.1200122

10 somatic interventions explained. (n.d.). Integrative Psychotherapy & Trauma Treatment. https://integrativepsych.co/new-blog/somatic-therapy-explained-methods

Therapy for cognitive & behavioral improvement. (2021, June 6). Brain Harmony. https://www.brainharmony.com/blog/2021/6/5/15-ways-to-create-vagal-regulation-at-home

Trauma Geek. (2023, February 9). *A neurodivergent review of the safe and sound protocol.* Medium. https://autietraumageek.medium.com/a-neurodivergent-review-of-the-safe-and-sound-protocol-84e5bc9120bf

Tsachor, R. P., & Shafir, T. (2017). A somatic movement approach to fostering emotional resiliency through laban movement analysis. *Frontiers in Human Neuroscience, 11.* https://doi.org/10.3389/fnhum.2017.00410

Understand trauma and the nervous system. (2023, April 12). Orchestrate Healthcare. https://www.orchestratehealth.com/understanding-trauma-and-the-nervous-system-an-interconnected-web/

Vago, D. R., & Silbersweig, D. A. (2012). Self-awareness, self-regulation, and self-transcendence (S-ART): A framework for understanding the neurobiological mechanisms of mindfulness. *Frontiers in Human Neuroscience, 6*(6). https://doi.org/10.3389/fnhum.2012.00296

van der Kolk, B. (2014). *The body keeps the score: brain, mind, and body in the healing of trauma.* Viking. https://ia601604.us.archive.org/35/items/the-body-keeps-the-score-pdf/The-Body-Keeps-the-Score-PDF.pdf

Vancampfort, D., Vansteelandt, K., Scheewe, T., Probst, M., Knapen, J., De Herdt, A., & De Hert, M. (2012). Yoga in schizophrenia: A systematic review of randomised controlled trials. *Acta Psychiatrica Scandinavica, 126*(1), 12–20. https://doi.org/10.1111/j.1600-0447.2012.01865.x

Walsh, K. (2018, October 14). *Developmental trauma "acts of triumph."* Karolina Walsh Psychotherapy. https://www.karolinawalsh.com/blog/2018/10/14/056-developmental-trauma-acts-of-triumph

Weibel, R. P., Kerr, J. I., Naegelin, M., Ferrario, A., Schinazi, V. R., La Marca, R., Hoelscher, C., Nater, U. M., & von Wangenheim, F. (2023). Virtual reality-supported biofeedback for stress management: Beneficial effects on heart rate variability and user experience. *Computers in Human Behavior, 141*, 107607. https://doi.org/10.1016/j.chb.2022.107607

What is Polyvagal Theory. (2024). Polyvagal Institute. https://www.polyvagalinstitute.org/whatispolyvagaltheory

The wheel of awareness instructions. (n.d.). University of the Free States. https://www.ufs.ac.za/docs/default-source/hr-staff-wellness-/wheel-of-awareness-activity.pdf?sfvrsn=852d9521_0

White, M. P., Alcock, I., Grellier, J., Wheeler, B. W., Hartig, T., Warber, S. L., Bone, A., Depledge, M. H., & Fleming, L. E. (2019). Spending at least 120 minutes a week in nature is associated with good health and wellbeing. *Scientific Reports, 9*(1). https://doi.org/10.1038/s41598-019-44097-3

Wong, S., Fabiano, N., Luu, B., Seo, C., Gupta, A., Kim, H. K., Shorr, R., Jones, B. D. M., Mak, M. S. B., & Husain, M. I. (2024). The effect of weighted blankets on sleep quality and mental health symptoms in people with psychiatric disorders in inpatient and outpatient settings: A systematic review and meta-analysis. *Journal of Psychiatric Research, 179*, 286–294. https://doi.org/10.1016/j.jpsychires.2024.09.027

Wright, A. (2022). *What is the window of tolerance, and why is it so important?* Psychology Today. https://www.psychologytoday.com/intl/blog/making-the-whole-beautiful/202205/what-is-the-window-of-tolerance-and-why-is-it-so-important

Zaccaro, A., Piarulli, A., Laurino, M., Garbella, E., Menicucci, D., Neri, B., & Gemignani, A. (2018). How breath-control can change your life: A systematic review on psycho-physiological correlates of slow breathing. *Frontiers in Human Neuroscience, 12*(353), 1–16. https://doi.org/10.3389/fnhum.2018.00353

www.ingramcontent.com/pod-product-compliance
Lightning Source LLC
Chambersburg PA
CBHW020529080526
44583CB00013B/791